I0103047

Stop and Reverse
Type 2 Diabetes

The Safe, Natural Method to
Improving Your Condition

Stephen Forbess, DC, DACBN, DCBCN, CCN

Copyright © 2015 Dr. Stephen Forbess.
No part of this document or the related files may be reproduced or transmitted in any form, by any means
(electronic, photocopying, recording, or otherwise) without the prior written permission of the publisher.

Cover Art Permissions.
Icons by Aha-Soft.com and Sara Carr Designs.
"Cherry Valley National Wildlife Refuge (Revisit)"
by Nicholas A Tonelli on flickr com.
Used with permission under Creative Commons license.

To my family, without whose time sacrifice and unending support, this work would not be possible.

Table of Contents

Who is Dr. Forbess?

The first chapters in books are usually reserved for other information, however my wife noticed that I didn't inform you, the reader, who I am, and what brings me to write this book. So here we go!

I always wanted to help people. And, I've been interested in the subject of good health through better nutrition most of my life. I recall my first contact with how nutritional products could help was in my teens. I had severe allergies, just like my father and my uncle. It was a common hay fever like condition, complete with excessive sinus drainage, sneezing and so on when I was around any pollen or cut grass. At that time my parents and I were involved with Shaklee© products, which had a very good educational program associated with their supplement line of products. I learned quite a bit about good nutrition. We encountered a nutritionist who evaluated me and recommended the Shaklee© alfalfa product and several other Shaklee©

supplements.   Within 3 months I no longer had allergies! By the way, to those of you familiar with Shaklee®, I find it interesting on my choice of career as a chiropractor and nutritionist, considering Dr. Forrest C. Shaklee, the founder of Shaklee® products almost 60 years ago, was also a chiropractor and nutritionist!

At any rate, at the age of 19 I decided to become a chiropractor. I earned a Bachelor of Nutrition Science (BS) and a Doctorate of Chiropractic (DC) during those early years. During my first 15 years in practice I went for additional training and earned a Diplomate from the American Chiropractic Association's Council on Nutrition (DACBN). I also earned a Certified Clinical Nutritionist (CCN) certification from the prestigious American and International Board of Certified Clinical Nutritionists organization. Several years later I took a Diplomate from the American Clinical Board of Nutrition (DACBN). Most recently I gained another Diplomate from the Chiropractic Board of Clinical Nutrition (DCBCN).

Needless to say, I have a high interest in nutrition! I have worked and helped thousands of people in the course of almost 30 years in practice, to improve and resolve their health conditions with both better nutrition and chiropractic.

Why Diabetes as a first book? I have a family history of type 2 Diabetes, beginning with my grandmother. My father also developed the same condition, and within 6 months of beginning nutritional changes I recommended, he was no longer considered a diabetic! Sadly, I never had the chance to help my grandmother. However, now I can help you!

Type 2 Diabetes is one of the most easily helped condition in our time. Its cause is connected to most of the top ten causes of death. Ridding ourselves of it will lead to improving life and living to those who pursue improved health, as described in this book.

Read and do as I describe below, and receive a reward... Improved Health and Vitality!

Dr. Stephen W. Forbess

xii

Introduction

Diabetes in today's "modern" society is mostly a condition of excess. Our society's diet and lifestyle causes the body to be so far out of balance, that conditions like Diabetes is the result.

Stopping and reversing type 2 diabetes is dependent on not only improving diet and lifestyle, but also rehabilitating the damaged organs that cause Diabetes. Hypoglycemia is the precursor to Diabetes, and most hypoglycemics or pre-diabetic individuals will find that making the changes discussed in this book will help them as well. This will reduce their likelihood of developing Diabetes from a "probability" to "highly unlikely."

Current conventional and traditional care consists primarily of diabetic medications by mouth or injection. Virtually no traditional treatment of the disease is coupled with a correction of the underlying cause or to rehabilitating the sick or diseased organ(s). With diabetes, giving medication without correcting the underlying problem is like giving children all the answers to their school tests. They would learn nothing, and consequently they would be deficient later in life when they need that knowledge. Simply giving drugs causes the doctor to be an enabler, with the medicated person becoming dependent on the drugs and never free from the disease. This creates an addictive person who thinks they have made the right choice, the only choice, and that there are no consequences to taking the drugs.

And what is even worse is that this 'epic experiment' on our society not only creates addiction, but it also causes other sicknesses, diseases, pains and disability. This may be either directly from the use of the drugs, or indirectly from a lack of attention to the central core cause of the disease. The underlying cause of most type 2 diabetes, if left uncorrected, will cause many to have conditions such as heart disease, liver disease, colon and digestive disorders, and cancer, to list a few.

Diabetes is the 7th leading cause of death. It is worse in minorities, with it being the 4th or 5th leading cause of death in those populations. And what is even worse, the underlying cause of most diabetic conditions, directly or indirectly causes or contributes to 7 out of the top 10 causes of death, including the leading cause of death, heart disease. These are all confirmed not only by my words, but in many published research journals. There is even a NEW diagnosis which connects some of these, which will be sure to add even more medications, called Metabolic Syndrome.

Again, correcting the cause, then rehabilitating the injured organs will give the body the opportunity to heal itself. Medications can eventually be greatly reduced or eliminated. With this, many diseases, conditions, and drug side effects could be avoided. You might be able to avoid being part of the top ten causes of death. Or put the conditions on hold for long enough that they may not bother you much or at all for the rest of your life.

So, ridding yourself of this cause could literally save your life. It will make you healthier, plus feel better and more energetic than you have ever felt. I am not kidding!

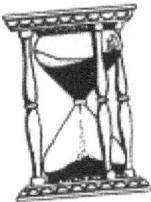

Time

There is a principle that states it takes time to get sick, and then therefore it takes time to get well. Stopping and reversing

Diabetes will take time, effort, and commitment. But the improvement you can expect will be well worth it. Most will see some initial positive changes within a matter of weeks. Being consistent with the changes recommended will ensure the best results.

Limitations of Matter

This is not a physics manual, however, there are limitations to the extent the body can naturally heal itself. Sometimes conditions have deteriorated and the body does not have enough time to complete the healing process. Fortunately, the vast majority of type 2 diabetics do not fall in this category. It is never too late to make the changes that the body can make use of to heal your body. I am continually amazed at how aggressive the body's amazing healing can be, when given the chance. These are best discussed with your Alternative Health Practitioner (see "Special Note - Your Team" in one of the next chapters).

The sooner you act, the better off you will be. I often tell my own patients, "If you wait too long to get your condition treated, there will come a point where not even myself nor Chiropractic nor Nutritional therapy will be able to help you." In other words, body organs will sometimes deteriorate to the point that they cannot repair themselves.

That being said, most of those with Type 2 Diabetes can stop and reverse this condition successfully. So, act NOW to help yourself!

What do you mean by Stopping & Reversing Diabetes?

Most people that use the proper tools, along with the recommendations given in this book, can successfully stop the continuing downward spiral of the Diabetic condition. They will find that they will reduce or eliminate medications directly associated with it. You should NOT stop taking related medication without professional assistance. If your doctor does not want to work cooperatively to decrease your medications as your condition improves and related testing (usually blood work) shows improvement, find another who will be willing to work with you (See chapter on The Basics). I am constantly amazed by the dogmatic belief of certain healthcare professionals that say, "once a diabetic, always a diabetic (type 2)," even in the face of positive changes in blood and other testing!

How To Use This Book

This book was written to help people, mostly on their own, to combat, fight, and win against type 2 diabetes! It can equally help those with hypoglycemia or pre-diabetes (type 2). You will learn about the necessary tools to make changes in your life. These changes will allow your body, and particularly your pancreas, to heal itself.

Your body was created with a wonderful ability to heal itself. This is often thwarted by man-made chemicals, poor diet, poor lifestyle, genetics, and many other factors in today's modern day society.

Pro-actively using this book will help stop and reverse type 2 diabetes, hypoglycemia, and pre-diabetes.

Follow the directions below to get the best results.

✓ First read the book completely. You will get a good understanding of what the repair process involves.

See me at my website at www.GoodNutrition.com for additional help, online training classes, webinars, supplements and other helps. We want to see you WELL!

✓ Support is important! Seek out an alternative health provider, such as a Nutrition Diplomate, Chiropractor with specialty degree in Nutrition, Certified Clinical Nutritionist, Naturopathic Physician, Alternative Medical Doctor, or other Alternative Health Practitioner (more on this in the chapter on The Basics). Choose someone who can give professional advice and assistance, as it is important to have a good support system.

✓ If you are under medical care for type 2 diabetes, ask your provider if they will be willing to work with you in this process. Specifically, *"As my condition improves based on blood testing, are you willing to reduce my diabetic medications?"* If they are not comfortable with this, find another medical or osteopathic doctor that will work with you (see The Basics chapter). Do not go through this process by yourself.

✓ If you are overweight, find a good health coach who is familiar with type 2 diabetes and will give you good support throughout the weight loss phase (as described later). Make sure they will help you transition to a healthy maintenance phase also.

✓   Eating the foods recommended are helpful and necessary to helping your body heal. Eat them!

✓   Supplements give your body essential nutrients that it needs to repair and heal itself. Take at least the basics recommended. Consult with an Alternative Health Practitioner (see The Basics chapter) to see if you need other nutrients as well. Supplements are concentrated substances. Don't take too many supplements each day. In most circumstances, I hesitate before giving anyone more than 4 different types of supplements daily. Some people's ability to breakdown or digest concentrated supplements may be limited or difficult.

✓   Perform daily exercise (see the chapter on exercise). Start slow and gradually increase. Even 5 minutes several times daily can make a difference.

✓   The final chapter helps put it all together. Read it! Do it! Reaffirming your commitment, being consistent AND being persistent over time will give you the success you desire and better health!

I know that you will have lots of questions. To help and assist those serious about their health I have created e-course companions to this book with additional explanations and helps at www.GoodNutrition.com. There are free resources as well, so check it out! Additionally, I have live webinars to answer questions submitted to me. I also discuss additional topics helpful to those with these health conditions. In addition to the e-courses and live webinars, you will find that webinars are archived, so you can watch them at your leisure. There are added resources and notes you can print as well as audio versions for those on the go.

The Basics

Welcome! You have now entered the world of natural health and healing! As you read this book, there is a core belief I have that you need to know.

Your body has an extraordinary ability to heal itself, if given the proper chance.

There are many things that I have discovered that will improve that ability. There are a few things that I need to tell you first, so you will get the most out of this book.

Each time Diabetes is mentioned in this book it is relates **ONLY** to **Type 2 Diabetes,** and does not include nor imply any other form of Diabetes, such as Type I Diabetes (or very uncommon forms such as Nephrogenic Diabetes, etc.), unless I specifically refer to another form of Diabetes. Type 2 Diabetes is the MOST COMMON form of Diabetes. If you aren't sure what type Diabetes you have, ask your treating physician. Being that Hypoglycemia and pre-diabetes are different degrees of type 2 diabetes, most references in this book can help these conditions as well. Questions from those serious about helping their health in this regard can be submitted to me, please visit my website, www.GoodNutrition.com for details.

Always consult with your *Alternative Health Practitioner* (see Special Note 1 below) and *Treating Physician* (especially if you are taking medication of any type), before beginning changes described in this book. A good question to ask your MD or DO physician (if you are taking medication) would be, "If testing shows I am improving, will you reduce my medications?" If your physician is not willing to work with you to reduce medication *as your condition improves*, find one who will. Do NOT reduce or drop your medication(s) without professional guidance and improved blood sugar testing. For type 2 Diabetic using injectable insulin, you are already trained to respond and react to increases and decreases in blood sugar via blood glucose testing throughout the day.

As you begin the changes referred to in this book, you can expect to see changes. To those using injectable insulin and insulin pumps, it is not unusual to see increases and decreases in pancreatic function **while the pancreas is healing itself,** causing **low and high blood sugars.** Continue to check your blood glucose levels frequently through the day. If using insulin pumps, please make sure you check your blood sugars frequently throughout the day! Highs and lows are to be expected. These levels typically get more normal as the pancreas heals itself. Always stay in contact with your Alternative Health Practitioner and your Treating Physician who is prescribing your Diabetic medications.

If you have a known allergy to any food or supplement mentioned in this book, it is not for you! It is important to have someone who can identify these situations and help. See an Alternative Health Practitioner to recommend alternatives.

If you do happen to be sensitive to one food or supplement mentioned in this book, this does not mean you won't be able to help yourself. Speaking to your Alternative Health Practitioner will be very helpful in these circumstances. The body is a wondrous healing agent. Do the rest that you are able to and watch your body improve!

If you currently have a serious or life threatening illness, such as cancer, or recently had a heart attack, or other serious illness, see your illness related physician for advice.

I like analogies, as it often helps to make a point. My intent is to always give you a clear understanding of what is being discussed. For ages analogies have helped many people with the understanding of concepts.

Special Note - *Your Team*

I will occasionally refer to two categories of professional help, the *Alternative Health Practitioner*, and your *Treating Physician*. Below is who they are, what they can provide, and why I refer to them as such:

Alternative Health Practitioner (AHP)

This is a health care practitioner who may or may not be a doctor or physician as described below. But he/she should be someone who has had advanced training in health and nutrition in a way that promotes the body to heal itself. They will understand or can research to gain the understanding of the methods described in this book to help your body heal itself. That person may be a:

15

1. **Diplomate from the American Board of Clinical Nutrition (DACBN)** - a board of DC's (Doctor of Chiropractic), MD's (Medical Doctor), and DO's (Doctor of Osteopathy), who have taken advanced courses in nutrition with board examinations to qualify.

2. **Diplomate from the Chiropractic Board of Clinical Nutrition (DCBCN)** - a board of DC's (Doctor of Chiropractic) who have taken advanced courses in nutrition with board examinations to qualify.

3. A chiropractor with advanced training in nutrition.

4. **Alternative Medical Provider** - A Medical Doctor (MD) or Osteopathic Doctor (DO) who has additional training in things natural, such as the *Complementary and Alternative Medicine degree* (CAM).

5. **Certified Clinical Nutritionist (CCN)** - This person may or may not be a physician, but has taken additional course work and passed an examination from the *American and International Board of Certified Clinical Nutritionists*, a reputable organization.

6. **Homeopathic (DHom), Naturopathic (ND), or Oriental Medicine (DOM) Physician.**

These professionals may be able to assist you in the natural process of healing.

I have provided a resource list for finding support alternative health practitioners in *"Appendix E - Alternative Health Providers Links"*. Check it out!

Treating Physician

In the USA, this would be the MD or DO who has diagnosed and prescribed medication such as insulin, tablets, or other medication to medically stabilize your condition. I recommend you find a treating physician who indicates their willingness to work with you. Make sure that as your condition improves, they are willing to change or reduce your medications.

Special Note - *Healing*

No one can "cure" you. However, the body has a great ability to heal itself! Simple cuts will heal, even without antibiotic ointments and without stitches (not that I recommend not to do these if necessary). The point is, our body is a self healing structure. Sometimes we need things to give our body the tools to heal. If you develop scurvy, a medical condition, your body is deficient in Vitamin C. Eating oranges or other high Vitamin C food or supplement will give the body the tools necessary for self healing.

My aim in this book, is to help you, the reader, to give your body the necessary tools and resources, so that your body will do what it was designed to do... to heal itself!

First Things First

Although I know that many people reading this book may know a lot about Diabetes, some may be reading to help a loved one or for their own education. Please read the next section completely. Everyone well informed of their own condition will learn something new or at least refresh their understanding of the condition. As well, the keys to success with the condition are located in this section.

Some may have a good understanding of what diabetes is and how it developed, some don't. I want all of you to have some basics, so we will have a good baseline understanding of how to successfully stop and reverse the condition. Please don't skip over this section. I have tried to keep it simple, and use few technical terms. That way you can get a better understanding of how to help yourself.

The Pancreas

What does the pancreas do?

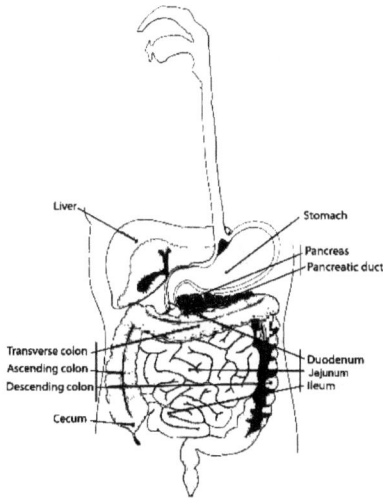

The pancreas is the only organ or tissue that produces insulin. Insulin "pushes" sugar into the cells of the body. Sugar gives the body energy. So the pancreas is an important organ. However, that is not the only function it serves. It also produces enzymes that are deposited into the digestive tract (intestine) that break down starches, sugars, fats, proteins, and acids.

Why are Enzymes Important?

Food does not get into the bloodstream and the body whole. It must be broken down into small pieces which are small enough to be transported into the blood stream. Enzymes are substances that help break down food.

When the pancreas is damaged, such as in the diabetic individual, not only is insulin production is affected, but digestion of the food may be impaired. This is one of the main reasons why many of those with Diabetes or Hypoglycemia also have digestive disorders and related problems. They have difficulty digesting foods, and incomplete digestion. As a result they miss out on key nutrients. Over time they may have nutrient deficiencies causing other conditions.

Why is Insulin important?

All the cells of the body need glucose or 'blood sugar' for a food/energy source. Insulin is the substance (hormone) made by the pancreas that "pushes" blood sugar into the cells. Too little insulin lowers energy in the body (see section on Hypoglycemia). Too much insulin (diabetes) will cause damage to the whole body, especially the nerves, kidneys, and eyes. Many diabetics suffer from diabetic retinopathy, loss of sight, heart disorders, lost sensation in place like the feet and hands (diabetic neuropathy), sores that do not heal, and so on. For some the damage progresses further, requiring kidney and pancreas transplants. Even these people can be helped.

5 Alarm Fire

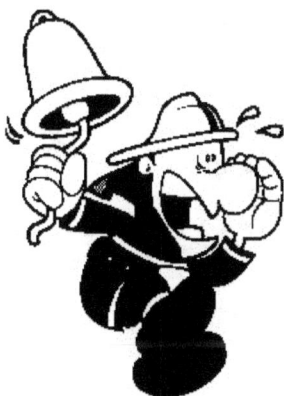

Any fireman knows that a five alarm fire will require lots of support and additional fire trucks. The same is true of the body. When we eat large amounts of starch and/or sugar, the pancreas signals a "5 alarm fire", and sends out large amounts of insulin to "mop up" all that sugar. When this is repeated frequently, day after day, at some point, the pancreas begins to get tired, and doesn't send enough insulin. As a result, a great deal of sugar stays in the blood stream. Blood tests will detect high amounts of sugar. Changes in lifestyle, discussed later in the book, can stop and reverse this!

What is Diabetes?

Causes of type 2 Diabetes is usually related to poor diet and/or lack of exercise. But at its core, type 2 Diabetes is a condition where the pancreas no longer works effectively. The pancreas is damaged. Insulin is a substance made in the pancreas. It "pushes" blood sugar (glucose) into the cells of the body. In diabetes, very little or no insulin is produced by the pancreas, resulting in very high blood sugar levels. What insulin is produced is low quality. This low quality insulin, even in higher quantities, doesn't do a good job of pushing sugar into the cells.

Some of the symptoms of Diabetes include (but not limited to): fatigue, nausea, frequent urination, excess thirst, blurred vision, frequent infections, loss of feeling in the feet and hands (numbness), and sores that do not heal. As Hypoglycemia is the precursor to Diabetes, symptoms of Hypoglycemia may also be found in the individual with Diabetes. More symptoms are listed in the section on Hypoglycemia.

I find it interesting to note that many Diabetics have digestive problems that are often undiagnosed. They may also suffer with seemingly "unrelated" with symptoms such as "poor digestion", excess gas, bloating, constipation, or diarrhea. Most find these symptoms are worse after eating "certain foods." With time, many diabetics or pre-diabetics will develop other symptoms, and they are often on additional medications for these conditions. As a result of making the changes recommended in this book, you may notice improvements here and require less medication as a result!

Normally when you eat foods that contain sugar, sensors in the mouth, stomach, and intestines activate. They tell the digestive organs to begin digestion. When starches and sugars are converted into glucose (the most simple sugar) they enter the blood stream. Other sensors tell the pancreas to produce insulin. The insulin produced should be proportional to the amount of sugar in the blood stream. Insulin transports the glucose sugar into the cells. As glucose is the main quick energy food for the cells, often we can feel a "lift" eating sugar. Problems occur when, over a period of months and years, we frequently eat high amounts of these starches and sugars.

What is Hypoglycemia?

Hypoglycemia is what happens **BEFORE** most people develop diabetes. It is the first step every diabetic went through, whether they knew it or not. In high school, college, and older ages, it is responsible for the afternoon tiredness many experience. Hypoglycemia is *Low Blood Sugar*. With these individuals, low blood sugar happens with increasing frequency. Many find temporary help from caffeine products, candy bars, or sugary treats to stay awake. High sugar and starch based foods actually worsen the condition, leading eventually to diabetes. It also affects their ability to learn.

In Hypoglycemia, the pancreas is **stressed** because we eat too much starch and too much sugar in the diet. Mental stress is a factor as well. As a result of high sugar and starch in the diet, the pancreas produces too much insulin. This large amount of insulin removes or "mops up" too much blood sugar causing low blood sugar, so we feel tired. Many of you may experience afternoon tiredness, the afternoon "blues", which is a result of low blood sugar. Over time this lifestyle puts high stress on the pancreas, causing damage. The pancreas loses its ability to handle blood sugar effectively.

Common symptoms of hypoglycemia are: fatigue/tiredness, anxiety, headaches, difficult concentrating, sweaty palms, shakiness, excessive hunger, drowsiness, abdominal pain, depression. As hypoglycemia worsens, the person becomes a "pre-diabetic". However, as odd as it sounds, many with hypoglycemia may not notice any symptoms at all! To their surprise the pancreas continues to deteriorate. Then on a routine blood test, high blood sugar (diabetes or pre-diabetes) is found!

What is Pre-Diabetes?

As hypoglycemia worsens, blood sugar levels vary wildly. There are still times of low blood sugar, but now there are times of high blood sugar, when the pancreas gets "tired". The pancreas is continuing its downward spiral of tiredness and sickness. The pancreas produces less and less insulin. The insulin it produces is lower quality, making it less effective to mop up blood sugar. It is tired and sick. **This is the pre-diabetic condition.**

Soon the pancreas will no longer make enough insulin to take care of sugars and starches from the diet. The pancreas spirals to an advanced stage of organ breakdown. Once it can no longer reduce blood sugar, the person becomes a full blown diabetic. By this time many but not all gain weight and fat from the excess dietary sugar, starches, and fats as well. Body fat often gets deposited where we see it, but also creates a fatty pancreas and heart, causing greater damage. If excess alcohol (lots of carbohydrates in alcohol) is consumed, the liver becomes fatty as well. Virtually every part of the body can and will begin to add fat. However, as odd as it may sound, many may not notice enough tiredness to concern them. Some experience no symptoms at all in this phase! High blood sugar is often the first signal of pancreatic problems and diabetes.

What About Genetics?

Many say they have or will get Diabetes because it's in their family. Not necessarily so!! Diabetes is a disease of excess for most. Genetically we all have strengths and weakness. A weakness, genetically speaking, does not generally mean you will get Diabetes. However, years living in an environment of eating too many starches and sugars, coupled with poor nutrient intake and lack of exercise, increases the likelihood of developing Diabetes with one who has this genetic weakness.

As another example, many smokers point to people with long lives who smoked all their lives cancer free. However, research shows that most of us do NOT have a genetic strength in this area. If you don't smoke, you have a very low risk of getting lung cancer. If you do smoke, you have a high risk of developing lung cancer. So being in the wrong "environment" of these dietary excesses will be harmful.

So, it is NOT a foregone conclusion that a family history of Diabetes means you are doomed to get it. Most can avoid Diabetes by taking precautions and doing the right things. Genetically speaking, some may have greater or less hunger, greater or lesser insulin resistance (insulin resistance is how well or how poorly the insulin in your body moves blood sugar into the cells), and some have a stronger or weaker pancreas (this relates to how fast the pancreas gets worn out -how much stamina and endurance it has). However, just like a coach who turns a weak athlete into a strong one, you can create a strong pancreas from a weak one!

Pancreas Function

Monitoring Pancreas Function

How do I tell how bad my sugar problem is, and when it is improved? How can I check my progress? How will I know when my condition is well or greatly improved? How long will it take?

These are good questions, and ones most people want to and should know. There are some good tests out there, and I will explain the common ones, as well as the ones I use to gauge improvement.

Blood Glucose

You get this in one of two ways. The most common is when you get a blood test. If the ordering doctor requests a "Blood Glucose" test or serum glucose, this is what is ordered. Another way is common to many, using the finger pin prick test. These are the testing kits you can do at home, and know the results right away.

Blood glucose is a measurement of your blood sugar at the time of testing. So if you ate a sugary meal, or had no food for 6 hours, this would influence the amount of sugar seen in this test. If your doctor orders a "Fasting Blood Glucose" at a laboratory, you should not eat after midnight and should get the test in the morning. (No eating for 6-8 hours)

Those doing finger prick glucose are getting a running total of glucose, not fasting, and are looking for high or low blood sugars, so they can inject themselves with appropriate amounts of various types of insulin. As any insulin dependent diabetic can tell you, this is not always successful. Often they have to inject larger amounts of insulin, or eat/drink sugary foods to try to normalize blood sugar levels so it doesn't get too high or too low. Out of control blood sugars can lead to a diabetic coma, and be very dangerous.

Anyone can obtain a blood sugar test kit from your local pharmacy to keep a check on their blood sugar.

Hemoglobin A1c (HbA1c)

This is a better way to detect diabetes. This test is not influenced by what you ate today or yesterday. The

HbA1c blood test evaluates hemoglobin in your red blood cells, and is a reflection of the average amounts of blood sugars over 2-3 months. This is a great test for assessing diabetes, and checking average blood sugar but not an effective test to see if the pancreas function is improving or not.

Glucose Tolerance Test (GTT)

This is the best test for pancreatic function. This is the test I recommend for hypoglycemics, pre-diabetics, and diabetics to determine when their condition is improving. I don't generally recommend it more than once every six months, and only if I they have been following through on the recommendations, as discussed later in this book, and see improvements in blood glucose and HbA1c levels.

Why is the GTT so important? This GTT test is a *functional* pancreas test. In other words, we are testing how well the pancreas is functioning *under pressure* to perform. As an analogy, lets say you are a runner who injured your hamstring muscles (thigh injury), and have trained for a 4K (4 kilometer) run, but have only trained with short runs, and been in the gym on treadmill, lifting weight, and aerobics classes. How will you know if your hamstring have healed and can run a full outdoor 4K? You would begin to run longer distances, putting pressure on the injured part to see if it is well, and see how well you do. It would be wise to do so a number of times prior to the race.

The Glucose Tolerance Test puts a load of sugar into the system and using blood tests, we can see how well the pancreas performs. Although not typically unsafe, insulin dependent diabetics may need to perform this in their doctors office, or in a lab facility.

In the GTT, you make sure you have fasted and have taken no diabetic medications, including insulin, since the night before (midnight). In a lab facility they will take an initial blood sugar test, then have you drink 100 grams of pure sugar (glucose). One half hour (30 minutes) after drinking the glucose, and then every hour for a total of six hours you will have blood sugar tests, for a total of about 8 blood sugar tests. Each test will assess how well the pancreas is managing blood sugar and how it reacts to moving that 100 grams of sugar out of the blood (insulin).

Full blown diabetes individuals will have very high blood sugars throughout all blood sugars taken. Some Diabetics will see blood sugars lower towards the end of the test. Pre-Diabetics will see blood sugars rise dramatically then fall closer to lower or normal levels. Hypoglycemics will see a rapid high blood sugar, then dropping to very low levels for the remaining blood sugars. Normally, blood sugars should rise to around 120, then drop to normal levels, as the pancreas is able to manage the glucose load. I typically place each blood reading on a graph, which makes it easier to evaluate, as well as compare to future GTT's.

The six hour GTT is important, as we need to see how the pancreas performs over time. Most doctors are only using singular blood sugar test and the HbA1c test. Some use the GTT, however usually only 2-3 hours. In order to see complete function, six hours is important. Especially when comparing multiple GTT's performed, 6 or more months in between. This lets the AHP and TP monitor changes, and when improvement is seen, reducing medication(for those who are taking them).

How Often Should I Get Tested?

Initially, as a baseline and for future comparison, I recommend one of each of the three tests. The 6-hour GTT is very important! If you are insulin dependent, continue your pin prick blood glucose test as your TP recommends.

HgA1c test -   This test should be performed every 3-4 months.

6-Hour GTT - If improvement is being seen on an abnormally high HgA1c test (1 full point or more), perform the GTT every 6 months. Some may see dramatic changes in the HgA1c levels. For some it may take longer, especially insulin dependent diabetics. Some may not have abnormally high HgA1c tests (hypoglycemics and pre-diabetics), so you should repeat the 6 hour GTT every six months. Your AHP can help determine improvement. Once your improvement levels off for 2 consecutive GTT's, your condition is stable. For most this means little or no medications! Always follow up with your treating physician (TP).

Coming Attractions!

Now that we have a basic understanding of type 2 Diabetes, lets move on to how most people can stop and reverse it!

For the remainder of this book, I will discuss changes that will need to be made in 5 areas. PLUS a section on how to put all of this together in one cohesive package. One chapter is dedicated to help the young, and stop and prevent future diabetics.

1. **Weight loss** - even one who is only a little overweight, losing weight and maintaining that lower weight, are components that are proven to be a major factors in diabetes reversal as well as maintenance of the well state. This leads to long-term results. Not all weight loss programs are healthy for diabetics. Different paths of weight loss will be discussed, as well as the better methods for diabetics.

– *SPECIAL NOTE* – If you are NOT overweight, never fear as most pancreatic healing for you will involve the other portions of the book. Please read over this section of the book anyway. Maybe you can help someone who is overweight!

2. **Diet** - In the section of diet, I will be write section on what to eat, what not to eat, and what foods will help the pancreas to improve and rehabilitate itself.

3. **Exercise** - Exercise is important, and helps to stabilize insulin and sugar.

4. **Supplements** - Food supplements are helpful as if taken properly (alternative health providers can help to guide you - see the next section). The pancreas needs specific nutrients to improve. Herbs and other supplements can help to improve and rehabilitate the pancreas. Pancreatic enzymes will be helpful with those having digestive issues.

5. **Professional Guidance** - As this is not the traditional approach, choose a *non-traditional guide.* Alternative health providers previously discussed in the Chapter on "Special Note - *Your Team*" can be important and vital. They can help determine the best combinations of all these factors you need. The right professional can help keep you accountable and on-

track. They can help set achievable goals, as well as recommending other changes to help. Also, it's not always a "direct flight" from point A to B. Sometimes you have "layovers." Different things need to be done at different times, especially if your condition is more complex, or if you have food allergies.

You are What You Eat!

What you eat is important! Just as some cars have trouble with low grade gas, your body doesn't perform well with low quality foods. I recall a car I had that began an engine pinging noise, indicating an engine problem developed by using a low grade gas. By switching to a higher grade gas I avoided the ping, and engine problems later on. **Your body is a highly developed engine, with specific nutritional needs. A quality diet is a must!**

Eating habits will be divided into several sections. I have included sections on specific foods to avoid, substitute sweeteners, and foods helpful to pancreas rehabilitation. Then we'll put it all together as to what a typical program should look like.

If you are overweight, know that weight loss is a vital component of this process and should be completed before making these changes. These changes will promote pancreatic healing, as well as helping to maintain your weight.

What to NOT Eat!

All healthy foods can be consumed in moderation. But for the Diabetic – Hypoglycemic – Pre-Diabetic individual, some foods should be temporarily avoided, limited or eliminated.

Starches

Starches are carbohydrates. On a food label, take the total carbohydrate grams, subtract any listed grams of fiber, sugar, and sugar alcohols (see the **Appendix D - Food Labels**). What is left, are probably starches. On a molecular level, starches are made up of many simple sugars that are "daisy chained" together. The more sugars are "daisy chained" together, the less sweet they taste. This is why starches do not usually taste sweet, unless mixed with simple sugars. Examples are pancakes (primarily a starch) with syrup (simple sugars), or sweet potatoes which is primarily starch, but naturally mixed with simple sugars (hence the name "sweet" potatoes).

The person with diabetes needs to clearly understand, **ALL STARCHES TURN INTO SUGAR!** The sugar that starches break down into <u>will</u> worsen their condition. This will not help their bottom line of stopping and reversing their condition. During the initial phase the **starches should be drastically reduced or eliminated.**

The body digests these "daisy-chained" sugars or starches and slowly breaks them down until they are simple sugars. The process usually takes 8-12 hours. This is why diabetics may eat a high starch meal like pizza or spaghetti in the evening may have a high blood sugar the morning after.

Processed Starches

These are the worst starches, as when they are processed they are pure starch. In nature there are no pure starch sources. Starches are found with minerals, vitamins, fiber, and other nutrients that help give the body a more balanced food source. Modern day processing removes most or all naturally occurring nutrient content. Man-made processing is performed because of cooking or baking needs/desires for certain textures (for example, soft bread). Processed starches come from grains such as wheat or rice. Important fiber and nutrients found in the outer portion of these grains are removed. The part used is the inner portion, which is made up almost exclusively of starch. This is the part that is mostly used for breads, pastas, and cereals.

Starch sources in ingredient labels include various flours, usually listed as white bleached or unbleached flour. Ingredient labels also show many ingredients with names ending in -ose, such as maltose, galactose, and so on. All these are starch or sugar ingredients. They have a specified length. When the digestion breaks down these into to the most simple sugars, they enter the blood stream almost simultaneously, or over a very short time, causing a sudden spike of blood sugar, stressing the pancreas further.

Food manufacturers take apart the grains, putting aside the healthy part like the "germ" and "bran," getting to the underlying starches. Most prepared grain products use a significant or high amount of this starchy "white flour" whether bleached or not. This starch is what gives us the consistency of bread or pasta to which we are accustomed.

By the way, food manufacturers don't throw away

the good "germ" and "bran" they take out of whole grains. The sell it to you again in products like rice bran, rice germ, wheat bran, wheat germ, bran flakes, and so on.

One last note on processed starches, as they relate to "sugar-free" products. Any sugar free breads, donuts, many candies, or other sugar free products usually contain high levels of starch! This means eating a "sugar-free" cake, **WILL PRODUCE LARGE AMOUNTS OF SUGAR!** This creates a sugar spike, about 8-12 hours later. This will not help achieving your bottom line of improving your overall condition.

Natural Starches

These are healthier starches, as they contain important nutrients essential for health. The starches are made up of different lengths of sugar, unlike processed starches. This allows a more gradual entry of sugars into the blood stream.

Some mistakes people make when eating natural starches, is not eating the skins of many of these foods. Potatoes contain many minerals and nutrients in the skins.

Natural starch sources also contain fiber, which has a beneficial effect on digestion. These are starches that are good to have in the diet once diabetes is stopped and reversed and the pancreas is healthy again.

However, during the initial phase while the pancreas is getting help, the person with diabetes also needs to understand that **even natural starches will all turn into sugar. Most natural, high starch foods should be avoided during the initial and rehabilitative phase.** Low starch vegetables are a better choice (See the Appendix on "Low Starch and Sugar Vegetables").

Sugars

Most know and have been educated in the harm of simple sugars in the diabetic condition. Don't be misled, **when you eat candies, cakes, donuts, chocolate, you are stressing and damaging your pancreas!** This will not help your bottom line of improving your condition. Some think that if you cheat with a candy bar or other sweet treat, you can simply take additional diabetic medications and have no consequences. Not so! The pancreas senses blood sugar and reacts, even if it is not able to produce enough insulin. Plus medications can have undesirable side effects, especially with frequent long term use. You will only cheat your results by doing so, and compromise your health.

Naturally occurring sugars in certain food groups, and in small quantities are acceptable. See the appendix section on "Low Starch and Sugar Vegetables". Grains may not have much sugar, however, are high in starches, previously discussed.

What about fruits? Generally, the only group fruits of acceptable one during rehabilitation also happen to be the highest nutrient-dense ones. I am speaking of the *berries*. These can be raw or frozen. This does not mean you can eat large quantities, but in small quantities, they are acceptable, and recommended. Generally, 2-4 of most berries daily is ok. Regarding natural or other sugars for those overweight, follow the guidelines in the chapter on weight loss until your weight is in acceptable ranges. Most other fruits are not acceptable and can derail your recovery and results.

Alcohol

Wine, beer, and alcohol consumption will affect blood sugar and the function of the pancreas. As well, many fermented foods and drinks contain alcohol as a result of the fermenting process and have similar effects. Alcohol from any source will affect diabetics with high and low blood sugars and increasing your appetite (not good if you need to lose weight). It will also affect the function of insulin and other diabetic medications, raise blood triglyceride levels and raise blood pressure. Additionally some will notice nausea, vomiting, a raise in heart rate, slurred speech and mental impairment when consumed in higher levels. Using alcoholic substances will limit or stop pancreas restoration and healing.

What about Red wine? While red wine has the health benefits of resveratrol and other antioxidants, the risk of worsening your diabetic condition outweighs the benefits. Resveratrol and other antioxidants can be obtained in supplement form if you desire.

Bottom line on alcohol use is that it should **not** be a part of your diet while diabetes still exists. **After the pancreas function has greatly improved or become normal**, if desired, alcohol can be consumed in limited quantities, and not more than one or two servings weekly. It's a good idea to talk to your alternative health practitioner about when you can safely put this back into your diet.

Starch & Sugar - The Bottom Line

Starches should be drastically reduced / eliminated. **Simple sugars** should be mostly eliminated during the pancreatic healing phase. For the diabetic most pancreatic healing / rehabilitation takes 2-5 years, depending on severity. If you need to lose weight, this phase of pancreatic healing begins once your weight loss is complete (once you've lost the weight you need to lose - see the chapter on weight loss).

Special considerations can be made for products designed to limit carbohydrate impact on blood sugar. Below are several that can be used, but in limited quantities!

Pasta

Many love pasta! However, whether whole grain or white pasta, the carbohydrate content is about the same. A typical serving size of pasta provides around 37 grams of starch (that means it will turn into 37 grams of sugar in the body!), and is unsafe for diabetics trying to allow the pancreas to rehabilitate itself. Enter *Dreamfields*© pasta. *Dreamfields*© uses a proprietary process that limits the effective grams of carbohydrates down to 5 grams per serving. They probably do this by adding an enzyme that temporarily blocks carbohydrate breakdown in the body's digestion. They also add a small amount of fiber which is beneficial. The limited effect on blood sugar has been confirmed by many diabetics online, who have tested their blood sugar, and found no sugar spike from carbohydrate digestion during 8-12 hours after eating. Limit quantities to 1 serving, no more than once or twice weekly.

PLEASE NOTE: All bodies are unique. Blocking the normal breakdown of starches may vary from person to person. If possible, check your blood sugars 8-12 hours after eating a serving of Dreamfields© pasta, and make sure your blood sugar does not rise. Eat a serving in the evening, and pay close attention to your blood sugar the next morning. If your blood sugar rises 8-12 hours after eating the this pasta, then you should avoid it. If you don't have the capability to check your blood sugars, then you should eat an evening meal of this pasta, then obtain a fasting blood sugar the morning after from your doctor. *Trust but verify!*

ADDITIONAL NOTE: It has been reported that leaving this pasta in combination with spaghetti sauce overnight destroys the carbohydrate blocking aspect to this pasta, so store uneaten cooked pasta separately from sauces. Pasta sauces have acids that probably, over time and in direct contact with the pasta, makes the carbohydrate blocking enzyme useless.

Side effects: I've noted none, except a positive effect with a few patients, that usually feel bloated after eating regular pasta. These people have noticed NO bloated sensations after eating Dreamfields©. For more information on their pasta product, as well as on their effect with Diabetics, go to their website at http://www.DreamFieldsFoods.com

Breads

Everyone seems to love bread! Sweet breads, sandwich breads, bagels, and so on. What to do?

Anatomy of a Wheat Kernel

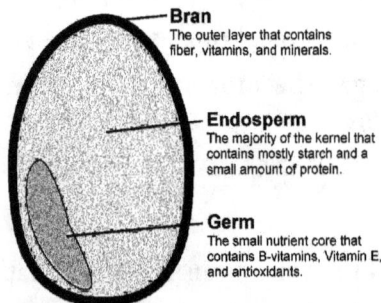

Bran
The outer layer that contains fiber, vitamins, and minerals.

Endosperm
The majority of the kernel that contains mostly starch and a small amount of protein.

Germ
The small nutrient core that contains B-vitamins, Vitamin E, and antioxidants.

ALL breads are filled with starch (endosperm of the wheat or other grain).

Whole grain versus white? A little secret, manufactures know you like SOFT bread. On the ingredient label the first ingredient of a whole grain product is usually the whole grain flour. BUT if you look further, note the next ingredient is probably some version of white flour, or starch added to help the loaf rise better. An authentic 100% whole grain bread with NO other type of flour will be very dense and hard. You can go to a healthfood store and look for this type of bread. It is usually smaller than a traditional loaf, dark in color, and very heavy, as this bread contains all of the grain (bran, fiber, and endosperm - see picture of wheat grain).

Needing to lose weight? Bread is OFF the list. If weight is not an issue, breads are allowed, but greatly limited. Make a sandwich with one slice of bread. Choose breads that are thin sliced. Used "diet breads" that have less starch / calories per slice. Only choose breads you like, since you are limited. Try "low carb" wraps, as the starches are very low. At the restaurants, if they serve bread at the table, have none, or tell them to not bring it if temptation is too great. I recall eating with the family at an Italian restaurant that did not serve garlic bread (I love good garlic bread). I had not had bread in a while and was looking forward to garlic bread. I decided that rather than waste my calories on the bread that was served, I chose not to have any. Several days later I had a garlic roll at my favorite restaurant.

The bottom line is that **ALL starch turns into sugar**. it is best to **avoid breads** during this process.

Sugar Alcohols: to or not to?

Sugar alcohols are substituted for sugars and similarly have a greatly reduced impact of sugar in the bloodstream. **They can have side effects** that include loose bowels or diarrhea, especially in those individuals with irritable bowel conditions. For most, when using small quantities, the body accustoms itself and loose bowels usually stop.

Those with bowel conditions should avoid these, although many find that small amounts (5-7 grams or less) do not cause digestive issues.

All should be cautious with foods having high quantities, as some protein bars I've seen have 15-25 grams of sugar alcohols. For those without bowel conditions, small amounts seem to be safe. *Listen to your body!*

Sweeten Your Appetite!

Discussions of sugars would not be complete without mentioning sweeteners, and my opinions of them. This is not an exhaustive study by any means, but I will discuss common sweeteners, as well as sugar-free sweeteners, and which ones I suggest using and why.

Common Sugar Based Sweeteners

Sugar based sweeteners are counter productive for the diabetic. They will worsen their condition, causing further damage to organs. Greatly limit, reduce or avoid these sweeteners. Look for them in foods on ingredient lists.

Sugar

Also called *cane sugar*, this is the sugar that has been around for thousands of years. **Avoid sugar!** This is the one to consume the least for a diabetic, although very small amounts are fine. These are found in most sweet things such as candies, sodas, sweet drinks, chocolate, and so on. These foods/desserts must be avoided.

Exceptions: Moderate to severe diabetics should follow the guidelines given by your treating physician regarding acute hypoglycemia and low blood sugar attacks. Drinking a high sugar drink or candy avoids a worse condition. *Be safe!* After you recover, continue on this process of self healing. Keep in mind that low blood sugars may be an indicator that the pancreas is beginning to function better! Over a period of time, as you see these things more frequently, you will give yourself less insulin, per your blood sugar readings.

High Fructose Corn Syrup

This is a very common sweetener, found in a variety of foods. It contains high amounts of sugar, in the form of a simple sugar called fructose. Fructose changes into glucose (blood sugar) and is readily absorbed into the blood stream, giving a sugar spike. Some claim this sweetener encourages an affinity or addiction to sweet things.

-ose Ingredients

Any ingredient ending in -ose is typically either a sugar, starch, or sugar alcohol. Sugars seen on labels include Glucose, Fructose, Maltose, to list a few. Starches (they convert to sugar - and are not usually a sweetener) include Dextrose and others. Sugar alcohols are a sweetener, but contribute very little to the blood sugar, and are better for the Diabetic, however can cause loose bowels or diarrhea in higher amounts. Pay close attention to food labels, as this will help differentiate the sugars, sugar alcohols, and fiber from other ingredients.

Agave Nectar

Many think this is a good alternative for diabetics. Not so! It is high in Fructose, which quickly converts to simple sugar in digestion. Look at the carbohydrates on the label. While this may be an option for non-diabetics, this is a no-no food for diabetics.

Sugar-Free or very low sugar alternative sweeteners

Aspartame (the "blue" label in restaurants)

Mostly under the brand Nutrasweet©. However in the ingredients you will find the chemical name "Aspartame". I've not been a fan of this substance, as since its introduction into our food stuffs in the 1980's there has been anecdotal evidence of health conditions from its use. I have had a significant number of patients that have had a wide range of negative side effects including headaches, depression, and simply not feeling well. I have found that simply eliminating aspartame from those individuals diet eliminates the side effects within days. Some investigations into aspartame use has found it associated with much more severe conditions. Aspartame is widely used in diet drinks, sodas, and sugar-free foods. If you have a concern with using it, searching online provides a wealth of information.

Sucralose - (the "yellow" label in restaurants)

This is a sugar-free sweet alternative chemical. Although I've not seen any real problems using this sweetener, I have read of anecdotal reactions. Some studies indicate a partial loss of intestinal bacteria, perhaps due to the chlorine ion in the product. Consumption of probiotics may help counter this effect. One study indicated a very temporary mild aberrant behavior of the blood sugar/insulin interaction, when both high amounts of sucralose and glucose was combined and taken all at once. Being that sucralose is used to substantially reduce or eliminate sugar in products, this reaction would not be a factor for most people. I would caution anyone combining a high sugar meal or snack, say several high sugar candy bars, with a highly sweetened sucralose-only sweetened drink. This is a sweetener that is probably OK for occasional use for those who do not have a known reaction to it.

Xylitol

This is a naturally occurring sugar alcohol. I've seen no problems with Xylitol, and it seems to have a beneficial effect on the teeth and gums, and has been shown to diminish cavities. It does have a small amount of carbohydrate content, so amounts need to be closely monitored if you are actively losing weight. Xylitol diminishes bacteria growth in the mouth so it has additional benefits. When someone is sick around our house, we use teas sweetened with Xylitol, for its health benefits in this area.

Saccharin (the "pink" label in restaurants)

Since the mid 1900's Saccharin has long been chastised within the nutritionist community with its possible carcinogenic (cancer causing) possibilities. More and more nutritionists are coming to an agreement that we are not seeing the types and rates of cancers related to its use. It may have been too much of an over-reach, however caution must always be taken with any chemical added to our foods. I don't see a problem with occasional use of this sweetener, in small quantities.

Acesulfame K

Acesulfame Potassium (K) is a non nutritive sweetener originally developed in Europe, has shown very few, or rare, side effects. I had one patient who had a severe side effect from use that included a red skin reaction, difficulty breathing, and had to be seen in a hospital. Anecdotal evidence of this type of reaction is rare. Often this is combined with other non-nutritive sweeteners. Diet Sprite is one product that uses this as the primary sweetener. If you have ever consumed diet Sprite, and not had a reaction, you probably will not have this rare side effect.

Herbal-based Sugar-Free or
Very Low Sugar Alternative Sweeteners

Stevia

An herb, when manufactured properly, made into a tea to make the extract, gives a sweet taste. Stevia is not sweet until processed. As it is much sweeter than sugar, it tends to have a bitter aftertaste like saccharin. Some brands combine Stevia with other things, including sugar, to diminish its aftertaste. Processed sweet Stevia is readily available in bulk, packets, and as a liquid water extract. If you buy raw stevia, you will have to process it yourself to obtain the sweetened variety. Truvia© uses stevia, combines it with erythritol, a sugar alcohol that does not seem to give and digestive issues, and has a product with very little if any bitter aftertaste.

Chicory root / Inulin

Under brand names like Just Like Sugar© and Sweet Fiber©, and sometimes, just as a listed ingredient, Chicory root tastes just like sugar, unlike stevia and saccharin, which are both about 100 times sweeter, and have bitter aftertastes. There is no bitter after taste PLUS there is naturally occurring fiber in the product.

What is my overall opinion of sweeteners?

I avoid Aspartame. When in restaurants and the like, and need a sweetener, I look for the yellow (Splenda) or pink (saccharin) stuff, take my own, or better yet, use none at all! Unsweetened tea can be very good! While at home I prefer Xylitol (a few calories), or Just Like Sugar® (chicory root). My wife likes Truvia® (Stevia + Erythritol - a sugar alcohol that does not have typical sugar alcohol side effects + natural flavorings). I think these are good alternatives. Although you will find sugar in our kitchen, it is rarely used. You can find your recipe needs for sweeteners can be accomplished with baking varieties of Truvia®, Splenda, or using Xylitol. All seem stable for cooking and baking needs. There are other manufacturers doing their own combinations of stevia or chicory root (inulin), and other ingredients. Look around and read the labels!

Size Matters!

Being overweight or obese can cause great damage to the person with Diabetes. Losing the additional weight takes pressure off not only the pancreas, but many other organs, including the heart, lungs, hips, knees, and ankles. An overweight person can not effectively reverse Diabetes. Excess fat is usable stored energy for the body. To remove it non-surgically, the body breaks fat down into . . .sugar! The problem is fat can be thought of as "compressed" energy. Gram for gram, fat represent TWICE the amount of calories than carbohydrates or proteins. This is one of the reasons fat is more difficult to reduce. It takes a lot more effort to reduce fat on the body.

Do I even Need to Lose Weight?

I have counseled Diabetics that were only 5-10 lbs

overweight, and told them how to eat differently to lose weight. The interesting thing is, once they lost those few pounds, they were NO LONGER considered DIABETIC, and no longer needed medication as a result. Weight matters!

Although every person is different, weight has a great impact on the normal body function.

There are several ways to calculate if you need to lose weight, BMI and Body Fat Analysis.

BMI

Basically a height/weight calculation, I've included a link to a chart below to calculate. Your BMI should be 20-24. Here is a link to one of my websites with a BMI calculator.

www.GoodNutrition.com

Although BMI is acceptable, a body fat calculator is a method that may give you a better way to get to optimum weight, because it is a device you place on the body, or hold with your hands or feet to determine the actual fat contained in your body. Purchase of one of these can give you a better idea of your fat weight, where a scale cannot differentiate between lean mass (muscle/bone), fat and water weight. Normal body fat for women is 18-24%, and men 15-19%.

Weight scales can be misleading at times. Muscle weight increases from exercise. Water weight may temporarily increase, perhaps due to eating too much salt, salty foods, or sodium. The weight scale alone can, mislead you to think you have not lost weight, when in fact you have. You won't see an extra pound of muscle, but that extra pound of muscle will burn hundreds of calories, even when you're sleeping, leading to faster weight loss and easier weight maintenance. Sadly it usually takes 2-3 months to build that extra muscle weight with most "couch potato" people, who aren't in the best shape.

If you find you are overweight/obese, either by BMI or body fat analysis, keep on reading below. If you are in the green zone and are at a good weight, great! Pay close attention to the rest of the book.

What about difficulties in weight loss?

Although there are many reasons people give for not being able to lose weight, I will discuss the two most common.

Thyroid

First are thyroid issues. Some blame weight gain on a faulty thyroid gland. Once most people with hypothyroidism (low thyroid) lose weight, find the thyroid improves as well. This may not be true with moderate or severe hypothyroidism. However, the person with any low thyroid problems, and have a overweight or obese condition WILL benefit from an improvement in diet.

Can low thyroid be helped with nutritional intervention? Yes, however special care is needed, overseen by an Alternative Health Practitioner, who has experience with hypothyroidism. Appropriate labwork will be necessary, to accurately be assured that the thyroid gland is healing itself.

Drugs and Medications

Second are drug interventions. Most weight gain from medications are related to steroid use. These cause a severe increase in blood sugar and weight gain is inevitable. For those requiring steroids for short term (1-2 weeks), began a weight loss program IMMEDIATELY following improvement of the illness being treated with the steroids. For those on long term or frequent drug use, seek the advice for weight loss from an alternative provider. If the drug treatment is related to a serious or life threatening illness such as cancer, you need to speak with the doctor who is prescribing the steroids to find out if and when it will be safe to begin a weight loss program.

Medically prescribed steroids will increase your weight, so be diligent about getting the weight off as soon as possible, after every episode of steroid intervention, so you can reduce pressure on the pancreas. Regarding the sick organs involved with drug use, seek care/advice from an alternative provider, as additional supplements may be helpful in improving the health of these organs, and may also help with the bottom line of reversing the Diabetic condition.

Losing the Weight

The Basics

Diabetes is a sugar related illness. Overweight individuals have high fat content. In order to lose weight effectively, the weight loss phase diet must be normal to high protein, low fat, low sugar, and low starch.

Some of the difficulties when losing weight is that often in many weight loss programs, muscle mass is lost. This can be damaging to the body and must be avoided.

I have found that people respond better, and stick with the program better in the weight loss phase if they lose weight faster, rather than slower. Some programs advocate a slower weight loss, say an average of 1 lbs weekly. The problem is the yo-yo effect this creates, as many find it difficult to stay on the program long enough to be effective. Then they frequently go on and off the weight loss portion of these weight loss diets. Yo-yo dieting is associated with eventually developing deficiency syndromes such as osteoporosis. This is bad.

Super fast weight loss (7-10 lbs weekly) may sound good, but has drawbacks. These programs include the medically supervised HCG diets (500 calories daily) and surgery related weight loss procedures. Learning how to maintain the weight is not a prominent feature of these programs. As a result, often these individuals gain the weight back, and then some, and they feel like a failure. These programs rarely teach people to eat properly. They are not taught the right foods and portion sizes, nor how to deal with the abundance of foods available in the stores or restaurants. With those that do encourage to eat healthier, this help rarely extends beyond the time it takes to lose the weight. This also creates the yo-yo dieting, with the consequences described above.

Safe weight loss is important. Getting all your vitamins, minerals, fiber, healthy fats is essential during the weight loss phase. Fad diets are short term weight loss (1-2 weeks) and what is lost is mostly water and muscle mass, which readily comes back on.

Weight loss *programs* are better, as they help, either through pre-designed foods, education, books, or a combination thereof. Programs help to keep a person more accountable.

Eating more frequently is better and teaches how to eat following the program for health and maintenance.

Weight Loss Programs

The programs I recommend for most Diabetics for the weight loss phase have an average weight loss between 2-5 lbs weekly, are low sugar and low starch, and emphasize healthy fats. Of the programs I have studied and recommended there are some that I come back to again and again when dealing with Diabetes. These are all **low sugar** and **low starch** programs.

Take Shape For Life

A Health coaching program that uses the Medifast prepared foods for most meals. Weight loss is faster for most than the other two programs mentioned below. Special programs are available for severe Diabetics, and those with certain other medical conditions. There are special programs for adolescents, teenagers, and seniors. Multiple university studies show safety and effectiveness (John Hopkins University). This is the lowest cost program of the ones discussed. There are no program or enrollment fees. The prepared meals are all low sugar, low starch, higher protein, low-fat foods. Contained within the prepared foods are 100% of 24 vitamins and minerals, including calcium, and 100% of your daily fiber. Included at no cost is a variety of live and online health coaching, for long term success. Live coaching is available with doctors, nurses and nutritionists, at no added cost. Educational books on diet and lifestyle are available. Many doctors use this program in their office, and can be overseen by them. Once you sign up, you can always receive free health coaching, listen and ask question on live calls for both weight loss and maintenance (the rest of your life) phases. Here is a link to our site more information on this program. My wife, Julie, is a health coach for the program, and this is her page.

http://drforbess4health.tsfl.com/

Atkins Diet

Another low sugar low starch program that is successful for diabetics. Books describe the diet. If you live near an Atkins diet center you can have the program overseen by a doctor. The books are relatively complete, although no personal coaching is available. You can use the program with good or bad fats. When using this program, I recommend using high quality choices and avoiding saturated fat and low nutrient foods. You will not learn as many of the essentials as you do with the Take Shape for Life program. However if you eat good foods, and follow the books, you will lose weight while keeping pressure off of the pancreas. Higher food costs and more preparation time are associated with this program.

Find books at Amazon about the diet. Go to Amazon.com and search for "Atkins" in their book category

www.Amazon.com

Or you can go to the Atkins website, where you can find more information:

http://www.Atkins.com/

South Beach Diet

This program is similar to Atkins with lower sugar and starch. No health coaching or professional support is given, other than what is written in the book. You can have good weight loss, though slower that either of the previous programs. Some of the differences, and the attraction for many on the South Beach Diet, is there are more fruits, starches, and sugars in the foods and prepared foods and bars recommended. You have to create a fine balance in order to lose weight. The extra starch and sugars may create difficulties for Diabetics. Blood sugar must be checked more frequently. If blood sugars are not cooperating, switch to one of the other programs above. Some of the prepared foods or bars may contain too many starches/sugars, so read labels carefully for starch grams. Higher food costs and more preparation time are associated with this program. I recommend one of the other two programs for most, as they are easier to follow, with higher success and greater ease to lose weight.

You can find books on the South Beach Diet at Amazon.com as well. Go to Amazon.com and search for "South Beach Diet" in their book category

Or go to their website:

http://www.southbeachdiet.com

Most other weight loss programs use too many starch grams to be effective for what Diabetics need.

Transition Phase after Weight Loss is the KEY to Successful Weight Loss

The most important time after losing weight, is the first year after weight loss. This should represent a "transition phase" when you are eating more appropriately, and not gaining weight back. With a properly designed transition period, some may continue to lose a few pounds. However some people end up "falling off the horse" and begin going back to their bad habits. Education and changing mindsets is key during this period.

Ideally you should have assistance of someone who can help you, and give advice. You would be well served using the services of a certified health coach. Such an individual can effectively help train someone to eat properly, watch portion and calorie size, and maintain weight. They can help you learn how to "eat to live" not "live to eat." This is essential, especially during the transition phase. Take Shape for Life will provide a certified health coach at no extra fee. If you are using one of the other programs, you can find a health coach in your area, or seek advice from an alternative health care provider.

How & When to Eat

This chapter is dedicated to those who have lost the weight they need to lose, and for those who do not need to lose weight. Everyone should read the weight loss chapter introduction (Size Matters) before this chapter, especially the section on how to determine if you are overweight. Whether you are only overweight by five or ten pounds, or two hundred fifty-five pounds, losing that weight might be the key to reversing your diabetic condition. DO IT!

The key to blood sugar is stability. How do you create stability? There are only two natural ways, through diet and through exercise. You need both. Exercise will be covered in a later chapter. The body is a highly developed complex engine that requires energy to work. By having a consistent energy source, your body will have consistent blood sugar. We receive energy through eating foods, that are broken down into small bits, that are then transported into the blood stream, causing an elevated blood sugar. Blood sugar elevating after meals is NORMAL. In diabetics this blood sugar is not transported very well from the blood stream into the cells of the body. So, the blood sugar collects in the blood stream, causing HIGH blood sugar. Often this is because we eat too much, or usually eat too many high sugar/starch foods over a lifetime.

So we need to eat smaller amounts, so we don't cause high blood sugars, just a slight rise in the blood sugar, which is normal. We'll talk about what to include in the meals later. In order to keep the blood sugar stable, we need to keep the blood sugar cycling through small rises and falls throughout the day.

How do we keep blood sugars stable?

Eating more frequently. Eating small amount of foods through the day helps give small rises of blood sugar, lowers hunger, allowing the individual to not experience the voracious hunger some feel when not having eaten for some hours. What's my point? **Eating frequently will stabilize blood sugar.**

How frequently?

The best information indicates eating 5-8 times daily is best. Most people fit into the 5-6 times daily. Most meals should be small in calorie content. 2-3 meals daily should be "snack" meals, typically 100-150 calories. Taller people will need a bit more, shorter will need less. Two or three times daily have larger meals, for example, eat more for breakfast and dinner times. Don't eat a large meal just prior to bedtime. Small meals/snacks should have very low sugar/starch content, low fat content, and higher protein content. Meals/snacks should be 2-3 hours apart, no more! If you are really hungry before the 2 hour mark, eat a little of another snack. It takes a few days to a week or two before you will accustom yourself to eating more frequently, less calorie foods. You should ALWAYS eat breakfast, as this begins the process of sugar stability.

A Typical 5-6 Meal Plan
Protein based, Low Starch, Low Sugar

Breakfast - Low-fat protein source, such as Eggs, or high fiber oatmeal or low starch/sugar protein bar.

Mid morning Snack - Protein based, low-fat snack

(100-150 calories).

Lunch - Salad or cooked vegetables with protein source.

Afternoon Snack - Protein based, low-fat snack (100-150 calories).

Supper/Dinner - Low-fat protein, Cooked vegetables or Salad, avoid starch foods.

After Dinner Snack - Protein based, low-fat snack (100-150 calories).

What TO eat!

When reading food labels, manufacturers seemingly hide a lot to when making a product they want us to like to eat. There are hidden starches and sugars. See my section on how to read labels, so you can avoid these pitfalls. So what should you eat? What kinds of nutrients should you take? What herbs are beneficial with diabetes? The next few chapters will discuss these. This chapter will go over some general topics that you should know with what to eat.

What makes the Pancreas different?

How does the pancreas differ from the heart, or the ovaries, or the glands? It produces something different than the others do. And just like a computer requires different raw materials to work that a steamroller, different body organs require a different makeup of

85

nutrients to make it run right and repair itself. Which nutrients? When reading a nutrition magazine or the newspaper, or looking online, you'll find hundreds or thousands of different formulas claiming to do this very thing. The pancreas is made up of millions of nutrients, and we've only struck the surface for what we know about them. There is no single magical nutrient that will "cure" it. Many of us are deficient in a number of nutrients, otherwise we would not have developed the condition. What specific help for one person may not help the next one. This is why I've developed a more broad-based approach, so to help the most people, within what can be achieved with diet and supplements.

We'll divide the nutrients into categories, and I'll suggest what I feel is the most important.

Whole foods

Foods are the best way to begin, as they have been shown for millennia to help many conditions. These are some of the commonly available pancreas building foods. I've also mentioned preparation tips that make these foods more appetizing.

Fresh or Frozen?

Fruits and vegetables find their way into the supermarket in both ways. When I first began studying nutrition over 30 years ago, I was taught "fresh is best". My opinion has changed, and for a very good reason. If you live on a farm, or own a fruit tree, or grow your own vegetables, when is the best time to pick fruits and vegetables, from a nutritional standpoint? When it is ripe! This is when the tree or vine has put the maximum final nutrients into these foods.

"Fresh" Fruits and vegetables

Consider the time it takes to get from the farmer to your supermarket. They plan for 10-12 days to get to market. What happens to ripe foods in 10-12 days? It goes bad. Now, what can the companies do to get it to you? They pick it while it is still green! Sometimes they use chemicals to "ripen" it, because they pick it so green. This is why, at times, when you eat fruit, it is tasteless. It is NOT tree ripened! So it also does not have all the best nutrients of tree ripened or vine ripened foods.

What about frozen foods?

Today, most companies wait to pick fruits and vegetables until they are ripe, and then bring portable "factories" to the fields where they grow them (especially fruits). They wash and freeze them when they are ripe! So most of your frozen foods are much closer to tree or vine ripened state. They will have more nutrient and taste value. This is better than "fresh" foods that are picked green. And often frozen varieties are less expensive as well. Sometimes, even considering this, some sugar is added to these frozen fruit varieties, as the tasters find they are not sweet enough. In looking at different batches from the same manufacturer, some have added sugar, and other batches do not. They add sugar at times to keep the taste of the fruits between batches consistent. They have to include this information in the ingredients list, so be sure to look.

Freezing foods does change the texture, especially for fruits, so fresh may make sense for some at times, such as adding blueberries to a salad, or eaten by themselves. However when making things such as a smoothie, or a sugar free jello, or other food where texture does not matter (unless you grow your own) use frozen. It's healthier!

Water and Fluids

There is no substitute for water. The body can tell the difference between coffee and pure water. That being said you should drink at least 8 glasses of water in addition to other drinks like coffee or tea. These other drinks do add to fluids on the body, but caffeine within them causes your kidneys to get rid of water, so drink more pure water!

Did you know that 55-60% of your body weight is water?

Water:

• MOVES nutrients, hormones, antibodies and oxygen through your body.

• REMOVES toxins & byproducts through the kidney & skin.

Even mild dehydration (several hours without drinking) affects your well-being, and will slow you down. You cannot STORE water in the body (and if you do, it's not healthy... ask anyone who has to take a diuretic drug). Daily you LOSE about 12 cups of water through perspiration (~2) and urine (~10), PLUS 2-4 cups through breathing, PLUS a cup through the soles of your feet! And, if you travel to a high altitude or a dry climate, you will lose even more.

The benefits of drinking water are many, such as:

- It's Calorie Free, yet helps keep you full!

- Keeps you from overeating (hunger can indicate mild dehydration)

- Removes TOXINS & WASTE

- Limits FATIGUE, HEADACHES

- Improves THOUGHT PROCESSES

- Speeds METABOLISM

Frequently people ask questions like these about water:

What's the best source for water? Plain, filtered water is best for quenching thirst... Plus it's cheap, calorie free, without sugar, caffeine or additives.

What about Distilled or Reverse Osmosis water? Minerals are removed from this type of water, so make sure to eat mineral rich foods or take a mineral supplement.

If I'm not thirsty, Do I still need to drink water? Thirst is a late warning on dehydration. Waiting for this symptom will slow you down, slow weight loss (if you are losing weight), and lower your body's ability to regulate itself well.

How do I know I'm not drinking enough? Tired feeling, hunger, headaches, darker than normal urine are all signs of dehydration. It's better to drink too much than too little!

Is it possible to drink too much water? Generally no. Exceptions are certain medical conditions (and you would be informed if it were) such as renal failure or congestive heart failure, or strenuous activity in a very hot environment. Don't drink more than 1 quart per hour. This gives your kidneys a chance to process all that water.

Drinking too little water allows toxins to build up, creating a "sewer" in your blood. It reminds me of when my children were very young and forgot to flush after using the toilet. By later that day or the next day, walking in that bathroom is horrible! How much more for your body. Your organs and tissues don't like to live in a sewer. Your body needs to flush itself, just like we flush the toilet. Bottom line is, you need to drink water to be toxic free, live well, and to achieve optimal health.

Pancreas building foods

This list of foods has various **beneficial effects** on the **health of the pancreas.** At least 2-3 of these should be eaten daily. Should you be allergic to any of these foods, DO NOT USE THEM. There are others to choose from. If you don't like a particular foods, rather than eliminate the food, try making it a different way. For example, with Kale, mix it fresh in a salad, cook it in a stir fry, or juice it and add it to a smoothie.

Berries - All the berries have a positive effect on the pancreas, and they are low in sugars! Berries are high in antioxidants, and are considered a nutrient dense food. Some berries such as Blackberries, Strawberries and Raspberries contain ellagic acid, which has shown beneficial for severe chronic conditions like cancer. Fresh or frozen. Don't go overboard! Use small amounts, 2-4 daily to limit sugars.

Green Tea - 1 cup several times daily.

Fresh Kale - a nutrient dense foods. Add to salads, or use steamed or lightly cooked. This foods is high in antioxidants, vitamin C and beta-carotene.

Arugula - another nutrient dense foods. Add to salads.

Garlic - great to add to many foods for flavor.

Onions - Limit quantities, as contains a small amount of sugars.

Spinach - Add to salads, scrambled eggs, or egg omelettes; or as a separate cooked side dish.

Red Reishi Mushrooms

Cabbage - Use in slaw, or lightly cooked or steamed.

Fish - Fish oils are important for many reason to the pancreas. Limit to once weekly, due to mercury content, and choose cold-water fish. Avoid swordfish (my favorite) as it has higher quantities of mercury.

Fresh Juice of mixed greens - kale, broccoli, spinach, etc... add to a flavored drink or down a 1/4 cup 3-4 times daily. Either purchase fresh at your local health food store, or consider purchase of a reputable vegetable juicer.

Supplements

These are **no substitute for eating the right way**, losing weight, or exercising. DO NOT use these by themselves. They work as a team, along with the other tools to achieve the goal of normal blood sugar and improved pancreas function. I rarely recommend a lifetime use of any special nutrient. The body should heal itself, and should not require the higher levels the repair process is complete. I typically recommend nutrients that aid the pancreas to be continued over a period of 2-5 years, depending on severity and the length of time one has had type 2 Diabetes. This gives the pancreas everything it needs during the complete process. Cells of the body turn over (are replaced) every 7 years (with a few exceptions). It is my intent to make sure the "next generation" of cells is healthier than the previous sick ones. In my online video course on Type 2 Diabetes, I discuss in more depth the supplements discussed below, and provide the ability for you to ask questions you may still have about them. If you are interested please see us at GoodNutrition.com.

In addition to any specific supplements listed below, it is important to take a quality **multivitamin-multimineral supplement** (NO Calcium) with meals, PLUS a **Calcium** supplement in a divided dose morning and evening. (Calcium is best taken away from meal times. Large amounts of calcium can block some nutrients from being absorbed, if taken at meal times)

Note on Iron sensitivities: Some iron-sensitive people may need to take iron separately from the multivitamin-multimineral supplement, and generally can be taken with calcium. If you think you are "allergic" to iron, know that most iron supplements are made from inorganic iron (iron from rocks, etc.) and some people have trouble with iron from rocks ("inorganic" source). "Organic iron" is iron taken from plants or other living organisms. Organic iron supplements are available from professional label nutrition companies (such as Standard Process) and may be available commercially as well in your health food store. Please also be aware that "organic" as in an "organic" iron supplement is not the same thing as "organic" foods you find in food stores. "Organic foods" reference the way and manner food sources are treated during growth. If you cannot find organic iron, contact me through my website, www.GoodNutrition.com, and perhaps we can help you obtain it.

Also, it is important for any supplement program to be overseen by an Alternative Health Practitioner (AHP), especially children, the elderly, and during pregnancy and breast-feeding moms.

Special Note on ALL Supplements: Whatever nutrient or nutrients are involved, quality is the most important thing you should have. For decades, nutritionists have warned people that poor quality vitamins, herbs, minerals and so on WILL NOT necessarily gain you the effects that you are attempting to achieve.

As far as vitamin extraction to make supplements, using a low heat extraction method has shown far better results in the human body than high heat methods. As the low heat method (-5 degrees Celsius) is a more expensive procedure, these supplements are usually more costly.

Herbs can be finicky when trying to cultivate them in a greenhouse environment, so some are still picked in the wild. Unscrupulous collectors of such herbs may combine the medicinal parts of the herbs with non medicinal parts, to make their "quota". *Standardized* herbs are herbs that have been independently evaluated, and supplemented with appropriate amounts of the medicinal parts to make a standardized amount.

All supplements are at risk by companies not subjecting their products to independent evaluations to at least verify what they say is in the product, IS IN THE PRODUCT. I recently saw in the news the name of some very public stores whose brand of supplements did not contain the nutrients stated on the label. I also recall a lecture given by a doctor several years ago, who determined that his patient needed iodine. However this patient stated his last doctor had made the same recommendation, so he went to a local store and bought iodine tablets. This doctor asked to see the supplement he had purchased, had the tablets evaluated, and found NO IODINE in the tablets. Independent evaluation (assay) is important, and only a few companies do it. Quality is KEY!

These are a few of the many reasons I recommend use *professional* lines of supplements and / or recommend *specific brands* of publicly available supplements. Although I could never check out every publicly available supplement company out there, out of the 100 or so companies I have checked I can give an OK to Nature's Plus©, KAL©, and Solgar©.

Interesting... If you ever open a Nature's Plus© product, it will contain a shrunk down copy of their latest independent assay of that particular supplement. They have done this for many years. Hats off to them!

Glandulars

Native peoples from all over the world usually ate the whole animal, not just the muscle, as we usually do in the U.S. When they have adequate amounts of food, these native peoples are usually healthier and live longer than the average.

Studies find that nutrients from glands and organs somehow find their way into the similar gland or organ of humans when eaten. Radioisotopes were attached to nutrients in the animal tissues, and were followed to where they ended up in the human body when eaten. Organ specific nutrients seem to have a beneficial effect on those types of organs in our body, so it is helpful to take them.

Glandular supplements are usually combined with other nutrients. Usually they are organs extracted from organic animals, put into tablet/capsule form so we can take them this way.

Look for supplements with glandular pancreas, usually bovine pancreas glandulars. These can be consumed daily, around ½ - 1 g daily, or more if approved by your alternative health care provider.

Specific Nutrients

Below is alist of helpful vitamins and minerals in diabetes. This is not an exhaustive search, and neither is it for every diabetic. Some are more helpful in pancreatic healing. Some are more helpful depending on the severity (affecting other organs or systems, such as the nervous system, eyes or kidney). I never recommend everyone taking all of these in high quantities, outside of what might be find in a daily multiple vitamin-mineral supplement. The top ones for most people to take in higher quantities include specific B vitamins, Chromium, Magnesium, and Fish oils. I've included a some references, simply to show you that nutrients have been widely used and studied to help this condition.

B Complex vitamins, especially B1, B6, B12

"B vitamins alleviate indices of neuropathic pain in diabetic rats," Jolivalt CG, Mizisin LM, et al, Eur J Pharmacol, 2009; 612(1-3): 41-7.

Chromium

- 200 mcg daily

"Beneficial Effects of Chromium in People With Type 2 Diabetes, and Urinary Chromium Response to Glucose Load as a Possible Indicator of Status," Bahijri SMA, Mufti AMB, Biol Trace Elem Res, 2002;85:97-109.

Unsaturated Fatty Acids

- 1-2 capsules daily

"Dietary Unsaturated Fatty Acids in Type 2 Diabetes: Higher Levels of Postprandial Lipoprotein on a Linoleic Acid-Rich Sunflower Oil Diet Compared With an Oleic Acid-Rich Olive Oil Diet," Madigan C, Ryan M, Owens D, Collins P, Tomkin GH, Diabetes Care, October 2000;23(10):1472- 1477.

Homocysteine, Folic Acid

- Folic Acid 10-50 mg 3-4 times weekly

"Homocysteine, Folate, Methylenetetrahydrofolate Reductase Genotype and Vascular Morbidity in Diabetic Subjects," Kaye JM, Stanton KG, van Bockxmeer FM, et al, Clin Sci, 2002;102:631-637.

Lipoic Acid (antioxidant - neuralgia)

- amount varies, only if needed

> *"The Therapeutic Use of Lipoic Acid in Diabetes: A Current Perspective," Coleman MD, Eason RC, Bailey CJ, Environ Toxicol Pharmacol, 2001;10:167-172.*

Vitamin E

- 100-400 IU daily (more under care of AHP)

> *"Vitamin E and Platelet Eicosanoids in Diabetes Mellitus," Gisinger C, Watanabe J, Colwell JA, Prostaglandins Leukot Essent Fatty Acids, 1990;40:169-176.*

Fiber - Oat or Rice fiber

> *"Cereal fiber improves whole-body insulin sensitivity in overweight and obese women," Weickert MO, Mohlig M, et al, Diabetes Care, 2006; 29(4): 775-80. (*

> *"Effects of Stabilized Rice Bran, Its Soluble and Fiber Fractions on Blood Glucose Levels and Serum Lipid Parameters in Humans With Diabetes Mellitus Types I and II," Qureshi AA, Sami SA, Khan FA, J Nutr Biochem, 2002;13:175-187.*

Vitamin D

- 2,000 IU daily (or more under care of AHP)

"Intake of Vitamin D and Risk of Type 1 Diabetes: A Birth-Cohort Study," Hypponen E, Laara E, Reunanen A, et al, Lancet, November 3, 2001;358:1500-1503.

Zinc

- 50-75 mg daily

"Zinc and Diabetes Mellitus: Is There a Need of Zinc Supplementation in Diabetes Mellitus Patients?" Salgueiro MJ, Krebs N, Zubillaga MB, et al, Biol Trace Elem Res, 2001;81:215-228.

Antioxidant Enzymes: Catalase, Superoxide Dismutase, Glutathione peroxidase.

"Antioxidants, Diabetes and Endothelial Dysfunction," Laight DW, Carrier MJ, Anggard EE, Cardiovasc Res, 2000;47:457-464.

Omega-3&6 Fish Oils

- 1-2 capsules daily

Fish oil supplementation improves endothelial function in normoglycemic offspring of patients with type 2 diabetes, Rizza S, Lauro D, et al, Atherosclerosis, 2009 Mar 19

Vanadyl Sulfate

- 100 mg daily

"Vanadyl Sulfate Improves Hepatic and Muscle Insulin Sensitivity in Type 2 Diabetes," Cusi K, Cukier S, DeFronzo RA, et al, J Clin Endocrinol Metab, 2001;86(3):1410-1417.

Magnesium

- at least 500 mg daily, should be 2:1 ratio (Calcium:Magnesium)

"Magnesium in Diabetes Mellitus," de Valk HW, Netherlands J Med, 1999;54:139-146.

Nicotinamide (The other form of Niacin)

- 500 mg - 3,000 mg

"Safety of High-Dose Nicotinamide: A Review," Knip M, Douek IF, Moore WPT, et al, Diabetologia, 2000;43:1337-1345.

Nutrients - Overview

Generally, for most diabetics, I begin with a multi-vitamin/mineral supplement, calcium/magnesium supplement, extra chromium supplement, and fish or omega oil supplement. The professional line of supplements I use in my office have better combinations, so there are fewer supplements to take.

My opinion on brands publicly available in health food stores are down to three, Nature's Plus©, KAL©, or Solgar©.

Helpful Herbs

While I don't recommend taking lots of concentrates (supplement tablets), herbs can be very helpful in Diabetes. DO NOT try taking all of these herbs at the same time, and consult with your alternative health provider before using these herbs to achieve best effect. See my section after the herb list, as to what I find most people start with.

Gymnema sylvestre

- 200-400 mg, 2-3 times daily

- side effects include low blood sugar, **so use with permission of TP & AHP.** It may lower the needs for diabetic medications.

- It lowers sugar cravings, may improve pancreas cells to produce insulin, and lowers blood sugar.

> "A Novel Gymnema sylvestre extract stimulates insulin secretion from human islets in vivo and in vitro," Al-Romaiyan A, Liu B, et al, Phytotherapy Research, 2010.

Grape Seed Extract

- 300-600 mg for 4 weeks, then reassess need

> *"Effects of grape seed extract in Type 2 diabetic subjects at high cardiovascular risk: a double blind randomized placebo controlled trial examining metabolic markers, vascular tone, inflammation, oxidative stress and insulin sensitivity," Kar P, Laight D, et al, Diabetic Medicine, 2009; 26(5): 526-531.*

Salacia Oblonga Extract

- 480 mg with high sugar/starch meals

- Some may have gastrointestinal side effects including gas and diarrhea.

> *"Extract of Salacia oblonga lowers acute glycemia in patients with type 2 diabetes," Williams JA, Choe YS, et al, Am J Clin Nutr, 2007; 86(1): 124-130.*

> *"Salacia oblonga extract reduces postprandial glycemia following a solid, high-starch meal." Steve Hertzler, Matt Washam and Jennifer Williams. The FASEB Journal. 2007;21:832.9*

Green Tea Extract

- Supplement should supply 600 mg Catechins daily (label should contain information)

> *"Green tea extract ingestion, fat oxidation, and glucose tolerance in healthy humans," Venables MC, Hulston CJ, et al, Am J Clin Nutr, 2008; 87(3): 778-84.*

Cinnamon Bark Extract

- 1-6 gm daily

"Cinnamon in glycaemic control: Systematic review and meta analysis," Akilen R, Tsiami A, et al, Clin Nutr, 2012 May 12.

Silymarin

- 200 mg daily

"Silymarin as an adjunct to glibenclamide therapy improves long-term and postprandial glycemic control and body mass index in type 2 diabetes," Hussain SA, J Med Food, 2007; 10(3): 543-7.

Olive Leaf Extract

500 mg daily

"Olive (Olea europaea L.) Leaf Polyphenols Improve Insulin Sensitivity in Middle-Aged Overweight Men: A Randomized, Placebo-Controlled, Crossover Trial," de Bock M, Derraik JG, et al, PLoS One, 2013; 8(3): e57622.

Curcumin Extract

- 500 mg 2-3 times daily

"Curcumin Extract for Prevention of Type 2 Diabetes," Chuengsamarn S, Rattanamongkolgul S, et al, Diabetes Care, 2012 Jul 6

Herbs - Overview

Herbs are an important component of improving the health and function of your pancreas. However herbs should not be taken indefinitely! Consult with your alternative health provider for continued testing to establish when pancreas function is normalizing. Once pancreas function is back to normal, special herbs, and special supplements for that matter, should be discontinued. With most people I often start out using these, as they have the greatest overall effect:

- Gymnema sylvestre

- Curcumin

- Green Tea Extract

- Cinnamon

Often people have difficulty taking capsules, so here are alternative methods to consume:

- **Green tea *liquid extract*** can be easily added to your drink instead of as a capsule.

- **Cinnamon spice** (1- 1½ tsp) - I would buy from the spice section at your food store, once daily in a food or drink also instead of taking capsules.

Please consult with an alternative health provider prior and while taking these herbs and supplements. Although these typically have few if any side effects, there are always those with allergies or sensitivities to supplements. Be safe!

Good Pancreas Enzymes

As mentioned before, when the pancreas loses the ability to produce insulin, the pancreas may also lose some of the ability to produce enough enzymes to break down foods in the small intestines. This especially true with those who are or have been overweight or obese. The pancreas can get fatty, diminishing its total ability to work. **Enzymes help break down foods**. If you notice any gastrointestinal upset, odds are you have a disruption of normal digestion. As a result of this GI upset, other conditions are caused, such as food allergies, hiatal hernias, ulcers, polyps, diverticulitis, colitis, pancreatitis, as well as other even more severe illnesses and cancers. It's a good idea to add enzymes whenever you eat, while the pancreas is repairing itself.

There are three primary categories of enzyme that can be helpful. They are divided int enzymes the help the breaking down of carbohydrates, fats and proteins.

Pancreatic Lipase

- This enzyme breaks down fat.

Pancreatic Proteases including Trypsinogen, Chymotrypsinogen and Carboxypeptidase

- These break down proteins.

Pancreatic Amylase

- This enzyme breaks down starches and other carbohydrates into sugars

Consult with your alternative health care provider about the need to take enzymes. As they help digestion, they should be **taken with food**. Enzymes taken by mouth are usually include *ox bile,* and may include a breakdown of more individual enzymes. Make sure it includes some type of all three important enzymes: lipase, protease, and amylase. Choose a reputable brand. Ask your alternative health provider for their recommendations. Look for products that do not use fillers or excipients. I prefer capsules or uncoated tablets, as they are more easily usable by the body's digestive system.

Exercise

Exercising daily is a must! **Regular exercise helps <u>stabilize</u> insulin & sugar levels**. Exercise helps **improve your insulin resistance,** and allows your body to do a better job with the insulin it has. Insulin will more effectively move blood sugar into the cells. Exercise improves the *quality* of insulin in your body, so a little will go a long way, and **your pancreas will heal more rapidly!** Please consult with your health care professional before beginning any exercise program, especially if you are excessively overweight, or have a serious heart, lung or other serious health condition.

> *"Role of Exercise for Type 2 Diabetic Patient Management," Pigman HT, Gan DX, Krousel-Wood MA, South Med J, January 2002;95(1):72-77.*

I recommend several types of exercise, as there are important benefits to each.

Aerobic Exercise

Depending on your ability, this could be as simple as a **20-40 minute walk every day,** or it could be taking an **aerobics class.** These classes are great for aerobics training. Good classes include **yoga, pilates, spinning, kickboxing, martial arts,** and so on. Good aerobics sports include **handball, racquetball, tennis, soccer,** and **basketball.**

Not all exercise is for everybody. Find one that you can do *consistently!* Don't do too much at once. If it's been awhile since you have worked out, start off with less. For example, for a scheduled 1 hour class, for the first week do 20 minutes, then gradually increase until you can do the full hour. The worst situation is when you do too much, feel overly sore or injured, and don't continue to exercise. Take it slow!

The purpose of aerobics is to work the great majority of muscles in the body. For those who have difficulty with a 20 minute walk, try splitting it into 2 ten minute walks a day. **For those who cannot walk,** or have to stay in a **wheelchair,** there is a wonderful DVD set called *"Sit and be Fit"* by Mary Ann Wilson. You can order these on www.Amazon.com.

Muscle Strengthening /Building Exercises

These types of exercise can **ADD muscle mass**. Especially for the overweight or obese individual, adding some added muscle mass will burn calories more effectively. This allows you to burn more calories, even when you are at rest or asleep.

How does this work? When you add muscle mass, you body must *maintain* that extra muscle, and consequently **must *burn more calories*** to keep it maintained! Thus you can lose weight even when you are sleeping. It takes 2-3 months of consistent muscle building exercises to begin to see these benefits. Also, I'm not saying you need to spend the afternoon in the gym (unless you want to), but I am saying that 3 times weekly spent doing a few exercises, is well worth the effort. It will also help you maintain a lower weight when you transition off the weight loss phase, and are enjoying life.

I've included a few examples of several at-home muscle building exercises below if a gym use is not used. These are beginning exercises, and more should be added.

Useful, easy, and inexpensive weights, if you cannot obtain regular hand weights is bagged rice. It is not advisable to eat (starch), but you can find inexpensive bags of rice in the food store. It comes in 1, 2, 5, 10 pounds bags, that are easy to grab. Another easy option for 1-4 pounds of weight is a canned food item in each hand. 8 ounces equals 1 pound, 16 ounces equals 2 pounds, 32 ounces equals 4 pounds.

Biceps Exercise - Basically flex your arm at the elbow from waist level to shoulder level, while holding onto a weight in the hand.

Triceps Exercise - While holding a weight in your hand, rest your flexed elbow on a wall in front of your chest. The elbow should be flexed, with the fingers facing towards your face. Keep your elbow on the wall in front of you during the complete exercise. Straighten the completely flexed elbow until it touches the wall at or above head level.

Deep knee bends (not too deep) This exercise affects large muscles, so in the long run is one of the more beneficial exercises. Hold onto a chair while performing the exercises.

On all the above exercises, perform them starting out at 2-3 sets with 5-15 repetitions during each set, and increase slowly, adding a few repetitions and then additional sets every week, until you are at the maximum, and continue at that level. For those of you already in an exercise program, keep it up!

What about a personal trainer?

Personal trainers can be helpful, and will give you motivation to improve muscle strength and endurance. Personal trainers can take you to new levels. Choose a trainer appropriate to your physical shape. If you have not been physically active for years, choose someone that is OK with a slower pace. You wall want a health coach who has some age and experience. You want to achieve exercise goals, not create so much pain you don't want to return for more. Expect some soreness, but if the soreness prevents your from wanting to continue to exercise, ask if that coach can slow down the pace, or find another coach. Don't stop!

Video Games - Xbox Kinect© and Wii©

I like these movement based video games, as they involve the whole body movement, while enjoying a bit of fun playing baseball, throwing darts, or going down the rapids, in a river, jumping, or dancing. It's lots of fun to exercise! I personally prefer the Kinect© system, as you don't have to hold on to a controller, the Kinect© controller detects you. These are competitive as well, so you can easily exercise with more than one.

Control of the Pancreas

Diet, Lifestyle, Exercise and Supplements have been discussed in previous chapters to help give the pancreas nutrients that can help it to heal itself, however, if the controlling forces that coordinate pancreas function, repair, and healing are not working well, then the pancreas will not heal as it should. There are three body systems that control or affect the function of the pancreas. They are the blood, lymph, and nerve systems.

Blood System

Heart - The heart pumps life giving blood to the body. If the heart suffers, all systems of the body suffers. If you have a heart disorder, more than likely, you already have a number of other organs involved. Discuss with your AHP alternative methods of natural help. Perhaps a future book will discuss natural methods of improvement and healing of the heart.

Arteriosclerosis - Often, sugar related disorders may go hand in hand with plaquing of the arteries. In this common condition there is liver involvement, and cholesterol levels in the blood stream are high or out of balance. A future book is planned on this topic alone, as many people deal with this condition, and there are other at-home therapies that can be done to reverse this condition. Dietary and lifestyle changes from this book, can be helpful, even if you have this condition. With the right protocols, most people will find no need to continue medication for cholesterol, based on blood studies. Regarding type 2 diabetes, arteriosclerosis (high cholesterol) usually is not a major factor regarding function of the pancreas.

Lymph system

The lymph system is present in the pancreas, but does not seem to be involved with the part of the pancreas responsible for insulin production. The lymph system helps to carry fluids and waste away, especially in infections. It does not seem to be much of a controlling factor in the pancreas.

Nerve system

The nerve system consists of the brain, spinal cord, and peripheral nerves ("nerves"). The brain controls and coordinates all function of the body. The brain contacts the body through connectors ("wires") called nerves. The nerves carry signals from the brain to all the organs and tissues of the body. When a nerve is damaged or impaired, it malfunctions. Wherever these malfunctioning nerves go is negatively affected. For example, if you damage or cut the nerves to the heart, it will lose rhythm, and will fail to effectively pump blood to the body. Without the connection from the brain to the body (nerves), the body malfunctions.

Nerves going to the pancreas come through two regions. Some nerves come down through the skull, passing next to the top neck vertebrae ("C1"), and other nerves come down through the spinal cord, then out through vertebrae in the mid-back ("T5-9").

Nerves are living, and are influenced much like wires in your houses electrical system. In your house, bad connections and crimped wires lead to a loss of electrical function. This is much the same in the body. Severed (cut) nerves result in a total loss of function, whereas pressure on nerves due to conditions like "vertebral subluxations" or "vertebral misalignment" causes a loss of function ("dysfunction") in the body.

Vertebral subluxations or misalignments can occur in the mid-back or neck due to a variety of factors, including poor posture and injuries. Chiropractic adjustments help reduce or correct these misalignments.

The Winsor Autopsies

Henry Winsor, M.D. questioned the validity of the connections between misalignment of the spine, nerve pressure and organ dysfunction.. At the University of Pennsylvania he conducted three studies where he dissected a total of 75 human and 75 cat cadavers. He studied the diseases they had, and looked to see if there was a connection between spinal misalignment and diseases in the human and cats studied. Interestingly, he found a correlation in every case he studied! Three of the cases studied had pancreatic diseases, and all three were found to have "minor curvatures" or misalignment of the vertebrae between T5 and T9.[1] Although this study was conducted quite some time ago, no research conducted since that time has reversed these findings. Since that time, the medical profession abandoned interest in nerve pressure and related connections to organ disease, and instead pursued other avenues of disease treatment primarily through drug and surgical interventions.

Current research into conditions associated with this nerve pressure confirms that spinal adjustments improve them. For example, a recent case study of chiropractic adjustments with a diabetic patient, found blood glucose levels normal after one month of chiropractic adjustments. [2]

Osteopathic manipulations are similar to chiropractic adjustments. Some osteopathic doctors (D.O.) still perform spinal manipulation. Osteopathic journals, concerning the benefits of osteopathic manipulation, still mention improvements of pancreas disease by correction of spinal misalignment. [3]

Bottom Line

While I did originally state that the current epidemic of type 2 diabetes is a condition of excess, there may be individuals that will not have complete resolution without correction of these misalignments, if present. Nerve pressure, either at T5-9 (mid-back) or at C1 (upper neck) may negatively affect the normal healing process. Little or no pain in the spine does not necessarily mean there are no misalignments. Most nerves do not cause pain, but instead control body functions, like the pancreas.

On a personal note: As aforementioned, I have a family history of type 2 diabetes. When I was in college, as well as in my first years in practice, I would have episodes of tiredness from low blood sugars (hypoglycemia). Interestingly, I did not have mid-back pain. However, my chiropractor usually found T5-7 area out of alignment. I found that shortly after adjustments to this area, blood sugars normalized and tiredness left. During that time in my life, I came to see the tiredness I occasionally felt, as a sign of spinal misalignment (spinal "subluxation"), and a reason to get a spinal checkup.

Professionally, when I see an individual with type 2 diabetes or hypoglycemia, in addition to the recommendations in previous chapters, I always check their spine as well, and correct misalignment issues. Although adjustments (joint manipulation) are not a substitute for the other changes recommended in this book, I think it is wise to seek a chiropractic spinal evaluation to ensure that nerve pressure is not a factor in the healing of the pancreas. I want you to have the best outcome! Do I always see misalignments at C1, or T5-9? Frequently I do! We adjust the spine and move on to the other steps.

What about Osteopaths? If your Osteopathic doctor (D.O.) performs joint manipulation (most don't), then by all means have them give you a spinal checkup!

References

[1] Winsor, H. *"Sympathetic segmental disturbances--II. The evidence of the association, in dissected cadavers, of visceral disease with vertebrae deformities with the same sympathetic segments."* Medical Times, Nov. 1921, 49, pp. 267-271.

[2] Blum, C. *"Normalization of Blood and Urine Measures Following Reduction of Vertebral Subluxations in a Patient Diagnosed with Early Onset Diabetes Mellitus: A Case Study"* Journal of Vertebral Subluxation Research, December 7, 2006. Pages 1-6

[3] Howell, Joel D. (1999). *"The Paradox of Osteopathy"*. New England Journal of Medicine 341 (19): 1465–1468.

Parents, Are You Raising the Next Generation of Diabetics?

What about our kids?

For decades type 2 Diabetes was known as "Adult Onset Diabetes." People who had this type of diabetes did not develop it until they were in their late thirties or older. Bringing if forward to today, children are now developing type 2 Diabetes in extraordinary proportions. **Teens and adolescents are at high risk.** They can be helped!

Let me be very clear. I again remind that I am speaking of type 2 Diabetes. There is another type of diabetes that affect our young as well, namely Type 1or "Juvenile Onset" Diabetes.

Type 1 "Juvenile Onset" Diabetes

These kids are already insulin dependent, as their pancreas is severely affected. Although much of what is being discussed in this book can be *helpful* with type 1 diabetes, and may help prevent the worsening of type 1 diabetes, it probably won't eliminate the need for insulin. Many of the changes, especially in lifestyle, diet, and exercise, should be helpful in stabilizing and managing their condition. Not doing so may and probably will shorten their life and increase their likelihood of developing many of the advanced conditions associated with out-of-control diabetes.

Juveniles with type 2 Diabetes

What can be done? Stop and reverse the process, and let the body repair itself. Our kids can beat this process, but they need our help and assistance. The cause of the development of this age of developing diabetes is important and must be discussed. *Children make their decisions based on environment, or in other words, what they are exposed to.* I can name a few categories of important influences: Family, friends and peers, media exposure (TV, movies, internet, video games, Facebook, Twitter, and so on). Their may be other categories you may need to add. However, their most trusted help comes from you as their parent!

Even though this is a book more focused on adults, this age is where it begins! You can change your child's outcome, to a life *without* diabetes.

Monkey-See, Monkey-Do

Your children watch and mimic much about you. They look up and respect you. After all, you are probably the only parents they have ever known. They have known you probably longer than anyone else in their life. They want to believe you make good decisions, and they want to be like you. Even though often you may butt heads and disagree.

Through my years of helping families, I have seen many families often make it easy for kids to make the WRONG decisions. It is not unusual for one parent to be aiming for healthy eating, while the other is exhibiting poor eating choices. Often the wrong foods "taste better." Kids take the path of least resistance. It's tastier to eat fried or fatty foods, than a salad.

Example: I know a family including a dad, a mom, and a few children. The mom has been eating healthier, making better foods, including good vegetables, whole fruits, leaner meats, and watching portion control. The dad however is a "meat and potatoes" type of person, and chooses to skip the vegetables, and most of the fruits, eating lots of breads, and a bowl of ice cream in the evening. What do you think the kids food choices are? Finicky eaters that are more into satisfying their taste palate, rather than eating a balanced diet. Oh, and some the kids are getting very overweight at an early age. These children, taking their parents actions, think its OK to eat poorly, after all dad does it! This is the childlike mind. Oh yes they can learn to make better choices, once they are older, maybe after some serious health condition, but isn't it far better to have them grow up learning better ways? Moms and Dads need to get on board, so their children will have a better, more balanced life!

Let me give you an example in my life. My mom made most of our meals when I was young. She made a variety of good foods, including fresh vegetables and fruits, and modest portion size. My dad always ate what she prepared, and so did I. Some years later, as a young adult, I recall going to a cafeteria style restaurant where you could choose all your foods. I spotted a bowl of turnip greens (my mom made this a lot while I was young, and was and still is a favorite food of mine). I said to my dad, "why don't you get some of the greens, they look really good!" But my dad said he didn't care for any. When we finally sat to eat, as was our custom, we would often share some of what we chose with each other. After tasting the cooked greens, I said, "Dad, have some, they a really good!" My dad said he didn't like greens, but had only eaten them when I was young for me, so I wouldn't grow up with his shortcomings. Wow! Although a small thing, it taught me a lesson.

Sometimes as parents we need to sacrifice our wants or desires, so our children will have a better life!

My dad never grimaced, nor gave any indication he didn't like a healthy food when I was young. As a parent, I have my likes and desires, for example, I don't particularly care for tomatoes or certain berries. With berries like blackberries, I don't particularly like the feel of the seeds in my mouth or teeth. I eat them with some frequency, without grimacing for my children. They like both. And you know what... I have found that I have grown to like certain varieties of tomatoes, and have an easier time "liking" blackberries and other heavily seeded berries.

Children need **healthy foods**. They need to **eat frequently**. See the chapter on "What to Eat". They need three larger meals and three snacks. Avoid the easily available predominance of starchy snacks like crackers, chips, breads, pizza. Focus on higher protein, low carbohydrate snacks.

Make sure they get **higher quality fats**. Unsaturated fats in nuts, seeds, and fish will help them to be able to think more clearly, and do better in school.

Starchy foods and vegetables, high sugar drinks and foods, and saturated fats found in many fried or fatty foods will drag them down during the day, and make it more difficult to function. These can make them more "hyper" and or slow them down as well at times. **So avoid starch and sugar foods.**

Kids tend to be active, the younger they are, so sometimes simply changing their diet by eating 5-6 times daily, and avoiding the bad foods will take the weight off of the overweight kids. Special concern regarding proper growth has to be balanced with the need to lose weight to take pressure off of the pancreas.

Kids with high blood sugar (type 2 diabetes/pre-diabetic/hypoglycemic) usually respond faster than adults with the same condition. Consistency and maintenance are the key factors in better outcomes, as well as the monkey-see monkey-do parental responsibility.

Overweight Kids & Teens

This needs to be overseen by both their pediatrician and your Alternative Health Practitioner. Sizes and development of children vary, and you don't want a lack of good foods to stunt their normal good growth and development. But as well you want to insure that a blood sugar or potential diabetic condition is avoided or resolved. Weight loss is important in overweight kids and teens, but you want to be safe first! I have provided a free body mass index calculator for both kids and adults on my website, www.GoodNutrition.com. This can help point the direction to see if your child may be overweight.

Supplements... They need them too!

It is IMPORTANT to obtain a good age appropriate **multivitamin-multimineral supplement**. The brands I recommended have special formulations for children and teens. I usually recommend that once puberty has begun, use a teen formula. Choose from the brands discussed in the chapter on Supplements. Some kids still have a hard times swallowing tablets/capsules, so feel free to choose chewables or liquid supplements from the same name brands mentioned. Your Alternative Health Provider (AHP) can help with this as well.

What about specific nutrients, glandulars (pancreas), and herbs? Generally, I avoid these, as most kids do just fine by making the diet & exercise changes. However this is better handled by speaking to your AHP.

Exercise... Combine Fun with Fit!

Make sure, especially for the older adolescent/teen, that they are involved in an active sport or other activity. When I was a teen, I was in marching band. My kids are involved in dance, kickboxing, and karate. Some get involved in organized sports.

But here is a better option for kids spending lots of time indoors. Video games.... But not just any video games. Choose the XBOX© with Kinect©, or the Wii Fit©. These games can combine fun with fit, if introduced properly.

Video Games - The problem

Handheld gaming systems where you can just sit for

the game creates no exercise, except perhaps in the mind, hand eye coordination, and thumb control & strength. This is not good enough!

This is the way I introduced it into my family, and it works! I purchased an Xbox© with Kinect© system and bought ONLY Kinect© games. Other games require the handheld controller, while sitting looking at the screen. The Kinect© sensor demands you to be up and moving throughout the game. You jump, throw imaginary object, shift, dodge, run in place, dance and so on. The sensor "sees" your body movements and rate it giving you the score you get. This satisfies the competitive fun kids look for, and they really burn up some energy doing it (calorie burn)!

I've seen others buy BOTH Kinect© games and regular games, and in those instances, kids tend to **not** play the kinect© games much, giving none of exercise benefit. If you already have a system with both types of games, **consider "retiring" the non-kinect©, hand controller based games** for a few months , and allow your kids to get some fun.. And get fit!

Find and work with a good Pediatrician!

Finally, as I've already said, it is important to check

133

with your AHP and pediatrician about your children. One additional note about pediatricians. When choosing a pediatrician, ask **how open they are to working with your naturally, nutritional minded AHP**, and using natural methods to combat illness when determined appropriate. More and more pediatricians are open to changes in diet and exercise, as they know kids are at higher risk to develop hypoglycemia and diabetes than ever before. My wife and I interviewed three different pediatricians before choosing one for our children. It made a big difference to have someone either supporting natural methods, or at the very least not obstructing the use of natural methods to get good outcomes without using medications, when possible. Don't expect pediatricians to understand most supplements or herbal uses, as their specialty are medical and drug uses, not natural methods. **Be safe and consult with your AHP!**

Puttin' It All Together!

7-Step Natural Pancreas Self-Repair & Healing Overview

1. Get Professional Guidance

I've mentioned it before, but there are five individuals that may be helpful:

• **Treating Physician.** If diabetic and on medication, find a doctor that will agree to reduce/eliminate your medications as your condition improves according to what they see on lab testing (see chapter The Basics).

• **Alternative Health Provider** - An alternative health provider who can recommend natural helps to your condition, especially if you have other serious health conditions (see chapter on *Your Team* and Appendix E on finding one).

- **A health coach.** Someone who can help monitor progress weekly, especially if you are overweight.

- **A personal trainer.** One who can improve your muscular endurance, improving insulin resistance, and working calories off, keeping weight under control.

- **YOU.** The most important individual is you! No one else can do it for you. You are responsible for your health. Make it happen! You can do it!

2. Monitor Your Improvement!

Use lab testing to keep track of your progress. Don't forget to get a baseline for all the tests. Make a file that you keep to look at your progress! Keep your team (TP, AHP,...) informed of changes, if they don't already know. Encourage your TP to begin reducing medications as improvement shows up on testing. Be safe! See the chapter on **Pancreas Function** for lab tests to monitor.

3. Make Dietary Changes to stabilize blood sugar (and to lose weight if necessary)

I can't say it enough. **Frequent small meals help stabilize blood sugar**. A low starch/sugar diet places very few sugar grams into the bloodstream. Everyone should go back and refresh on the importance of avoiding starches & sugars, and review sugar alternatives

136

so go to these chapters to refresh:

<u>What to NOT Eat!</u>

<u>Sweeten Your Appetite!</u>

Overweight: If you are overweight by even a few pounds or obese, losing the weight is a big key to long term success. Use a program of weight loss. Support is important. Studies find that people are more successful in losing and keeping off the weight if they use a personal health coach to keep them accountable. Whatever program you use, get the weight off. Go back to these Chapters to refresh and begin your program, then proceed Normal Weight paragraph.

<u>Size Matters!</u>

<u>Losing the Weight</u>

Normal Weight: If not overweight, or if you have lost the weight, eat a low starch/sugar diet for at least 2 years, to give your pancreas breathing room to heal while doing the next two steps to help the pancreas to repair itself. Go back to these chapters to refresh and begin:

<u>How & When To Eat</u>

<u>What TO Eat!</u>

Pancreas Building Foods

I have more information related to foods later in this book:

Appendix A - Good High Protein Food Sources

Appendix B - Low Starch and Sugar Vegetables

Appendix C - Healthy Snacks

Appendix D - How to Read Food & Nutrition Labels

Also, there may be additional resources if you download the electronic version of this book. Updates to the eBook appendixes may be updated occasionally, and available if you re-download the book to your device. If you go to my website (listed several paragraphs below) and register your email, I will keep you updated as to what is available to you regarding additions, and if there is any charge for the same (there would probably be no charge if you re-download your ebook from where you purchased it online).

4. Exercise to tone muscles, improve insulin function, and lose/maintain weight.

Exercise does two helpful things in diabetes,

improves insulin resistance (insulin works better) and burns calories. AND it also helps to boost natural energy levels, improving moods, and helps the feeling of overall well-being. Perform a minimum of daily walking or swimming, and a minimum of 1-2 times weekly of something more aggressive, whether it be weights or sports, or exercise related video games as discussed. Read the chapter on Exercise.

5. Supplements to promote Pancreas healing

This is very important. Giving the pancreas the nutrients it needs, while at the same time being on a program of low starch/sugar, will give the pancreas the breathing room it needs to begin to repair itself. Remember that this process takes time, typically 2-5 years. Avoid supplements you have a negative reaction, or are allergic to. Look again at the chapter on supplements.

6. Get your spine checked for misalignments

You don't want to slow down your recovery. Correcting spinal misalignments that improve the function of the pancreas could speed your recovery.

It's a good idea to get a spinal checkup from a board certified chiropractor (DC) or osteopathic physician (DO) - verify the DO performs spinal checkups and manipulation, not all do. Read the chapter on Control of the Pancreas.

7. Check for Additional Resources and Natural help at my website, wwwGoodNutrition.com.

I do realize that this is a lot of information, things to do, and so on. It can be overwhelming. I have additional resources that can help many of you through the process. On my website I have a video e-course, based on this book, plus webinars where I can answer your questions. These webinars are live, but also are recorded and archived, so you can look to see if your question may have already been answered, and you can help yourself more readily. During the live webinars, I also do live teachings on various health topics to help you reach better health and enrich your life. Plus there are occasionally live or recorded interviews with movers & shakers in health or nutrition to give you additional perspectives on optimal health. Find out more at www.GoodNutrition.com.

Maintain a Healthy Pancreas!

Create a Lifestyle of Health

Realize that starch and sugary foods are your enemies. Keep starches like breads, pastas, pastries, pizza crusts, and so on at a minimum. Eat very little sugars. Occasionally for a week or two, go on a starch free, sugar free diet. Once monthly do a weight check. If you gain more than a few pounds, take a week or two to get the weight off. Continue to exercise daily and weekly as recommended.

And Finally, Follow My Success Formula

Commitment

+ Consistence

+ Persistence

+ Time

= Success!

Commitment

Agree with me to **begin** this process. Commit yourself to **finishing** this and **improving** your health.

Consistency

Consider the ant. It works consistently, day in, day out to accomplish its goals. Every day reassess your progress of eating, exercise, and supplementation. **Stay on track!**

Persistence

No one says it will be easy. Your lifestyle and eating habits created who you are. If you "fall off the horse" and eat something inappropriate, don't kick yourself. Get back up and start agin tomorrow.

Time

It took time to get here, it will take time to get back your health! A few months or several years is a small price to pay for a lifetime of good health.

!!! Success !!!

In the first days weeks and months, you will enjoy different measures of success. Many find improvements in their **energy**, sense of **well-being**, and **digestion**. As time goes on, more improvements and successes will follow. Blood sugars will go up and down as the pancreas has bouts of improved function. It may be like a car with bad gas that coughs and sputters, until it gets to the good gas. Pancreas function will be up and down. As blood sugars become more consistent, you will know it is improving. Following through with the recommendations in this book will increase your energy, and give you a new zeal for life!

Be in Health and
Enjoy the Rest of Your Life!

144

Appendix A - Good High Protein Food Sources

If losing weight, choose lowest fat sources. Nuts are not helpful during weight loss.

Lean meats & fish (4-7 ounces)

- Trim all visible fats

- Cook meats thoroughly and throw away grease, to keep fat content lower

- put meat on paper towels, especially with ground meats, after cooked to remove additional fat/oils

- Turkey and chicken tend to be lower in fat

- Eat skinless meat. Skins are very fatty.

- Avoid fried meats.

- Avoid fatty meats

- Cook meats via baking, broiling, or on a grill.

- Eat fish 1-2 times weekly, as fish oils are rich in the healthy omega fatty acids.

- Limit processed/deli meats, as these are often higher in fat, salt, and often contain hidden starches and sugars.

Nuts (small amounts - 8-10 nuts)

- Almonds are best, as they contain chromium

- Avoid higher fat nuts (macadamia or brazil)

- Avoid peanuts. They are not nuts, but are legumes, and their fats are not as healthy.

Soy / Tofu / Soybeans

- Try it! Not all soy tastes the same. Various brands have "tofu crumbles" and can be substituted for ground meat.

Cottage Cheese - low fat or fat free

- ½ to 1 cup satisfies the protein content for a typical meal.

Eggs

- if heart or cholesterol problems exist, use egg whites only.

- have no more than 4-7 eggs weekly.

Appendix B - Low Starch and Sugar Vegetables

While I cannot comment on every vegetable, these are common ones are best and more easily available. Always read labels for sugar and starch content. Highly colored (dark green, brightly colored yellow/green/red) are usually more nutrient dense, more nutritious, and for these reasons, better for you. Choose well!

Arugula	Eggplant
Asparagus	Endive
Bok Choy	Escarole
Broccoli	Fennel Bulb
Cabbage	Green or Wax Beans
Cauliflower	Hearts of Palm
Celery	Jalapeño
Collard/Mustard Greens	Jicama (Cooked)
Cooked Spinach	Kale
Cucumbers	

Kohlrabi

Lettuce (Green Leaf,
Butterhead, Iceberg,
Romaine),

Mustard Greens

Mushrooms

Nopales

Okra

Peppers (Any color)

Portabella Mushrooms

Radishes

Red Cabbage

Scallions (Raw)

Spaghetti Squash

Spinach (Fresh/raw)

Spring Mix Lettuces

Sprouts (Alfalfa &
Mung Bean)

Summer Squash
(Scallop, Zucchini,
Crookneck, or
Straightneck)

Swiss Chard

Tomatoes

Turnip Greens

Turnips

Watercress

Appendix C - Healthy Snacks

Usually these are meals 2, 4, 6 of the days. (Meals 1, 3, and 5 are what I consider Breakfast, Lunch and Dinner)

(These are <u>not</u> meant the weight loss phase for those that need to lose weight. See the chapter on weight loss)

This is by no means a complete list, so add your own! I look for foods or food combinations that are low calorie (150 calories or less), low starch, low or no sugar, and low fat. I also like to see more than 5 grams of protein, however that is not an absolute requirement. Avoid aspartame sweetened foods as much as possible! I am seeing more and more foods sweetened with OTHER alternative sweeteners, so look around! For example, I've noticed more and more low calorie Greek yogurts are being sweetened with stevia or sucralose, not aspartame, and that's better for you!

Vegetables

- 1 cup baby carrots

- 1 cup fresh broccoli, 1cup fresh cauliflower with 2 T low-fat or zero calorie ranch dressing

(*Zero calorie dressings?* Check out dressings made by Walden Farms (www.waldenfarms.com). Order some and find those that you like, and use it!)

- 2 cups raw spinach, 3/4 cup sliced cucumber, ½ cup cherry tomatoes, ½ cup chopped carrots, and 2 Tbsp balsamic vinegar

- 4-6 oz Chobani® or other brand **nonfat** **plain** **greek** yogurt or 4oz nonfat sugarfree yogurt

Nuts & Seeds

- 2 Tbsp sesame seeds

- 3 Brazil nuts

- 30 pistachios

- 3/4 oz trail mix (no fruit)

- 7 walnut halves

- 14 almonds

- 16 dry-roasted peanuts

- 3/4 cup edamame

- 1-1/2 oz low-fat mozzarella cheese

- Deviled egg: Cut 1 hard-boiled egg in half, mix

the yolk with 1 Tbsp hummus, and fill the egg white with the yolk mixture

Fruit & dairy

- ½ cup blueberries with 1/4 cup **nonfat plain greek** yogurt or nonfat **sugarfree** yogurt

- 1 cup fresh halved strawberries, ½ cup blueberries, and 2 Tbsp **Sugar Free** whipped topping

Fruit & protein

- ½ cup 1% low-fat cottage cheese with 5 medium strawberries or 1/4 cup blueberries

- ½ cup 1% low-fat cottage cheese and 4 large olives

Fruit & vegetable

- 1/4 cup pureed avocado, 1 Tbsp chopped tomatoes, 1 tsp lime juice

Vegetable & protein

- 1 medium tomato, sliced, sprinkled with 1 oz low-fat mozzarella cheese

- ½ cup 1% low-fat cottage cheese with ½ medium tomato, sliced

- 5 4-inch celery sticks with 1 Tbsp natural peanut butter or other nut butter

- 1 cup raw portabella mushrooms with 1 oz low-fat grated mozzarella cheese

- 1 cup sliced eggplant with 1 oz low-fat mozzarella cheese melted on top

- 3/4 oz tuna mixed with 1 tsp lemon juice and 1-2 tsp. Low fat mayonnaise and wrap in several romaine lettuce leaves.

- 1 cup chopped broccoli with a 1 cubic-inch square of cheddar cheese melted on top

- 8 cherry tomatoes with 1 cubic inch of cheddar cheese

- ½ cup sliced red bell pepper with 3 Tbsp hummus

- 3 fresh basil leaves, 1 medium tomato, sliced, and 3 Tbsp hummus

- 2 Tbsp hummus, 2 Tbsp avocado, and 3 large celery stalks

Nuts/seeds & vegetable

- 10 almonds and 3 large celery stalks

Protein & dairy

- 1 large egg scrambled with 1 Tbsp shredded cheddar cheese

Appendix D - How to Read Food & Nutrition Labels

How much "sugar" is in this food product?

According to food manufacturers, this sample food label would be considered "Diabetic friendly" simply because the "sugars" on the label are very low. However, this is not the case because of the high starch content (starch is turned into sugar in the body). Starch is not required to be listed on food labels. BUT it can be easily calculated.

Nutrition Facts		
Serving Size 1 Cups (1g)		
Serving Per Container 16		
Amount Per Serving		
Calories 240		Calories from Fat 54
		% Daily Values*
Total Fat 6g		**9%**
Saturated Fat 1g		**5%**
Trans Fat 0g		
Polyunsaturated Fat 2g		
Monounsaturated Fat 3g		
Cholesterol 0mg		**0%**
Potassium 25mg		**1%**
Sodium 125mg		**5%**
Total Carbohydrate 39g		**13%**
Dietary Fiber 9g		**36%**
Sugars 2g		
Sugar Alcohol 4g		
Protein 8g		**16%**
Vitamin A 10%	●	Vitamin C 4%
Calcium 30%	●	Iron 5%

*Percent Daily Values are based on a 2,000 calorie diet. Your Daily Values may be higher or lower depending on your calorie needs.

	Calories	2,000	2,500
Total Fat	Less than	65g	80g
Sat Fat	Less than	20g	25g
Cholesterol	Less than	300mg	300mg
Sodium	Less than	2400mg	2400mg
Total Carbohydrate		300g	375g
Dietary Fiber		25g	30g

155

How to calculate the amount of sugars that significantly affect blood sugar from a given food:

Total Carbohydrate

   - Dietary Fiber

    - Sugar Alcohols

= Net Carbohydrates affecting blood sugar

Example (based on graphic example)

  39g   **(Total Carbohydrate)**

- 9gm   (Dietary Fiber)

- 4gm   (Sugar Alcohols)

= 26gm (Net Carbohydrates affecting blood sugar)

AND

26gm of Net Carbohydrates affecting blood sugar

- 2 gms sugar (listed on label)

= 24 grams Starch ("hidden sugars")

According to the label example above, the 2 gms sugar listed as sugar on the package will get into the bloodstream within minutes to an hour (the time it takes the body to break down simple sugars into glucose)

The remaining "hidden sugars" (24 gms) will turn into blood sugar within 8-12 hours of eating it.

Sometimes the **"Nutrition Facts"** on smaller packages may be listed in a text format. So make sure you look for the breakdown of the Total Carbohydrates. There are not always fiber, sugar or sugar alcohols listed, and that is because they are either not present, or in quantities less that .5-1gm (when the quantity is so low, they may not be required to list it)

Appendix E - Alternative Health Providers links

Here are some links to help you find *your* Alternative Health Provider:

The American Clinical Board of Nutrition (ACBN) is a national certifying agency in nutrition. The ACBN is accredited by the *National Commission for Certifying Agencies* (NCCA). The ACBN offer Diplomate status (**DACBN**) to all professional doctors in the health care field, after qualified course work training (over 300 hours) and passing national board exams. Continuing education is required. Their Diplomate directory is below:

http://www.acbn.org/certificants.html

The Chiropractic Board of Clinical Nutrition (CBCN) is a credentialing and certifying agency that was formed as a chiropractic specialty board. The CBCN operates under the auspices of the American

Chiropractic Association (ACA. The CBCN awards a Diplomate (**DCBCN**) to Doctors of Chiropractic in the field of Clinical Nutrition, following qualified course work training (over 300 hours) and passing national board exams. Continuing education is required. Their Diplomate directory is below:

http://www.cbcn.us/diplomate-directory

Chiropractors with a high interest in nutrition (if they do not have a diplomate in nutrition) often have an advanced degree in nutrition or nutrition Science (B.S., M.S.,or PhD). They may have a separate professional degree in Naturopathy (N.D.), homeopathy (D.Hom.) or Oriental Medicine (D.O.M.). Often they may also be certified in acupuncture. The best way to research this is looking for a local chiropractor and looking on their website for more information.

Alternative Medical Doctor with an the *Complementary and Alternative Medicine degree* (**CAM**). There is no central organization that lists all current Medical providers with the CAM degree, however the *Academy of Integrative Medicine* has some listings of alternative minded medical providers. As above, check out that providers website to look for the CAM degree https://aihm.org/find-a-provider/ When searching on their site, pay special attention to the individual doctors area of expertise. There is the *American Holistic Nurses Association*. They may work with alternative medical providers, so you might look here as well.

http://www.ahna.org/Home/For-Consumers/Practitioner-Directory

The International & American Associations of Clinical Nutritionists organization is a reputable organization that teaches and trains individuals and doctors through a 300 hour course in nutrition. They award a certificate (**Certified Clinical Nutritionist - CCN**) on passing their board examination following successfully passing their course. This may be a healthcare professional, or a nutritionally minded individual (non-doctor). This is not a post graduate program, as this certification does not require a healthcare doctorate degree for the individual to take the course work and examination. All CCN's are to have at least a Bachelor of Science degree prior to being certified.

http://www.iaacn.org/

Homeopathic Physicians - There is no one organization that lists all homeopathic physicians, however these are a few to look through. Again, look at their websites, and call their office to ask if they work with Diabetes. Ask if they restrict themselves to homeopathic remedies only, or if they are more holistic and recommend whole foods and supplements (vitamin and herbs). You want a more holistic practitioner.

https://www.homeopathy.org/homeopaths-directory/registered-homeopaths-directory/

http://homeopathyusa.org/member-directory.html

http://www.homeopathycenter.org/find-homeopath

Naturopathic Physicians

These physicians are very knowledgeable about a variety of supplements and strategies to helping illness and disease.

American Association of Naturopathic Physicians. http://www.naturopathic.org/AF_MemberDirectory.asp?version=1

American Naturopathic Medical Certification Board - email this organization for a referral to an ND near you. information@anmcb.org

Doctor of Oriental Medicine

American Association of Acupuncture and Oriental Medicine

http://www.aaaomonline.org/search/custom.asp?id=320

National Certification Commision for Acupuncture and Oriental Medicine

http://mx.nccaom.org/FindAPractitioner.aspx

Stop and Reverse Type 2 Diabetes, Hypoglycemia, and Pre-Diabetes

© 2014 by Dr. Stephen Forbess. All rights reserved. No part of this book may be reproduced in any format without the permission in writing from the copyright holder. For further information, contact Dr. Forbess through www.goodnutrition.com.

www.ingramcontent.com/pod-product-compliance
Lightning Source LLC
Chambersburg PA
CBHW072145270326
41931CB00010B/1890